This is my Cancer Sucks Coloring Book

Color Test Page

Color Test Page

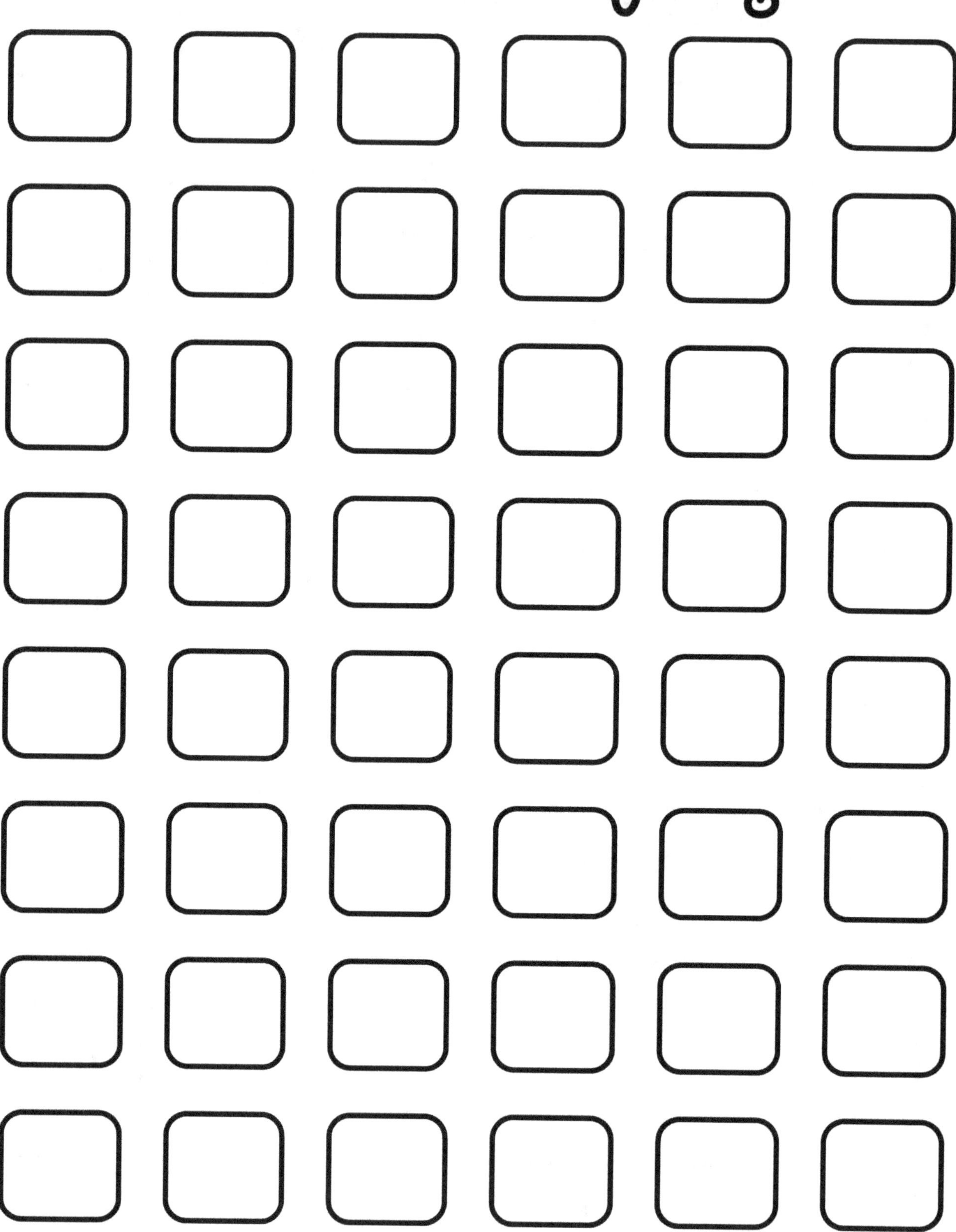

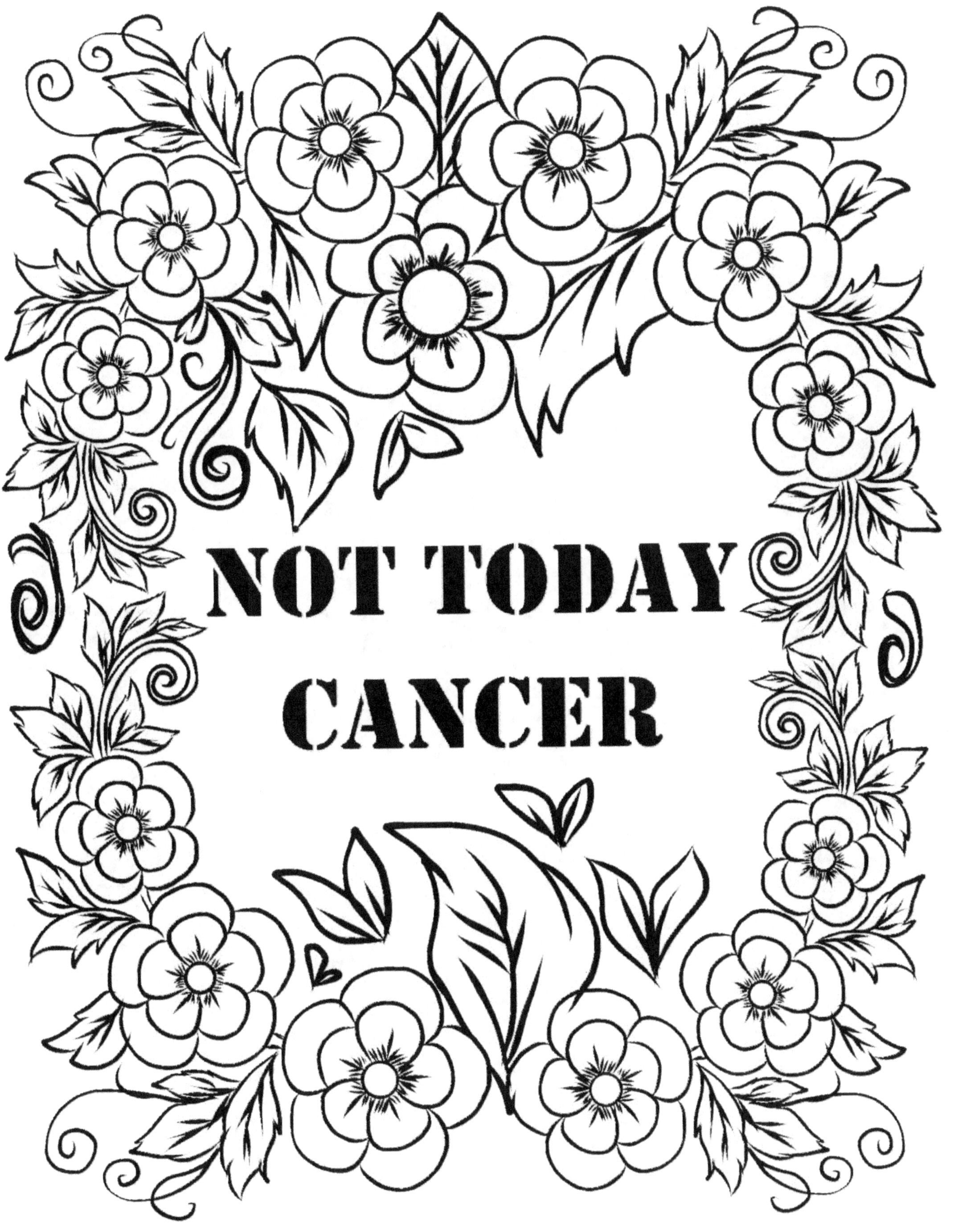

NOT TODAY
CANCER

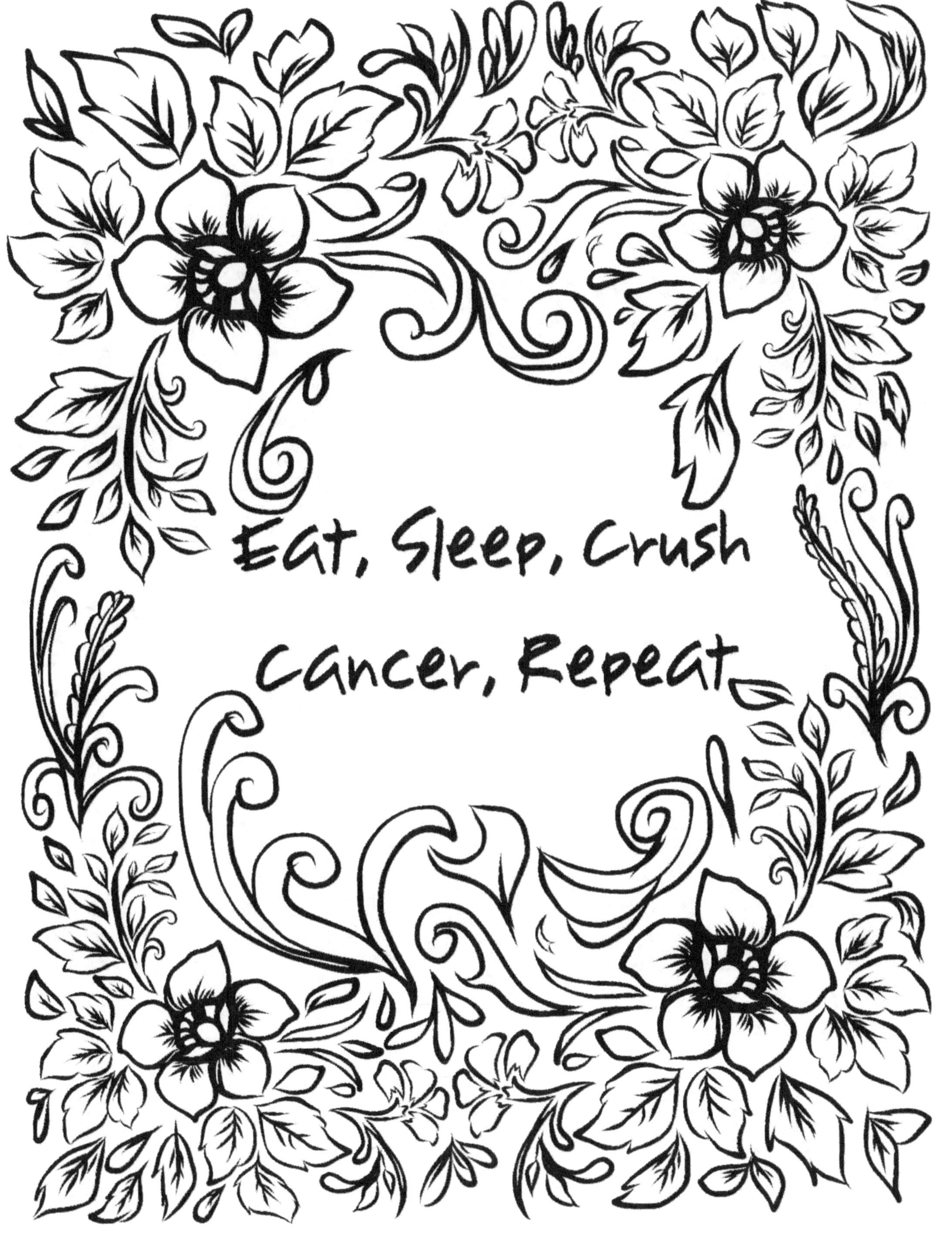
Eat, Sleep, Crush
Cancer, Repeat

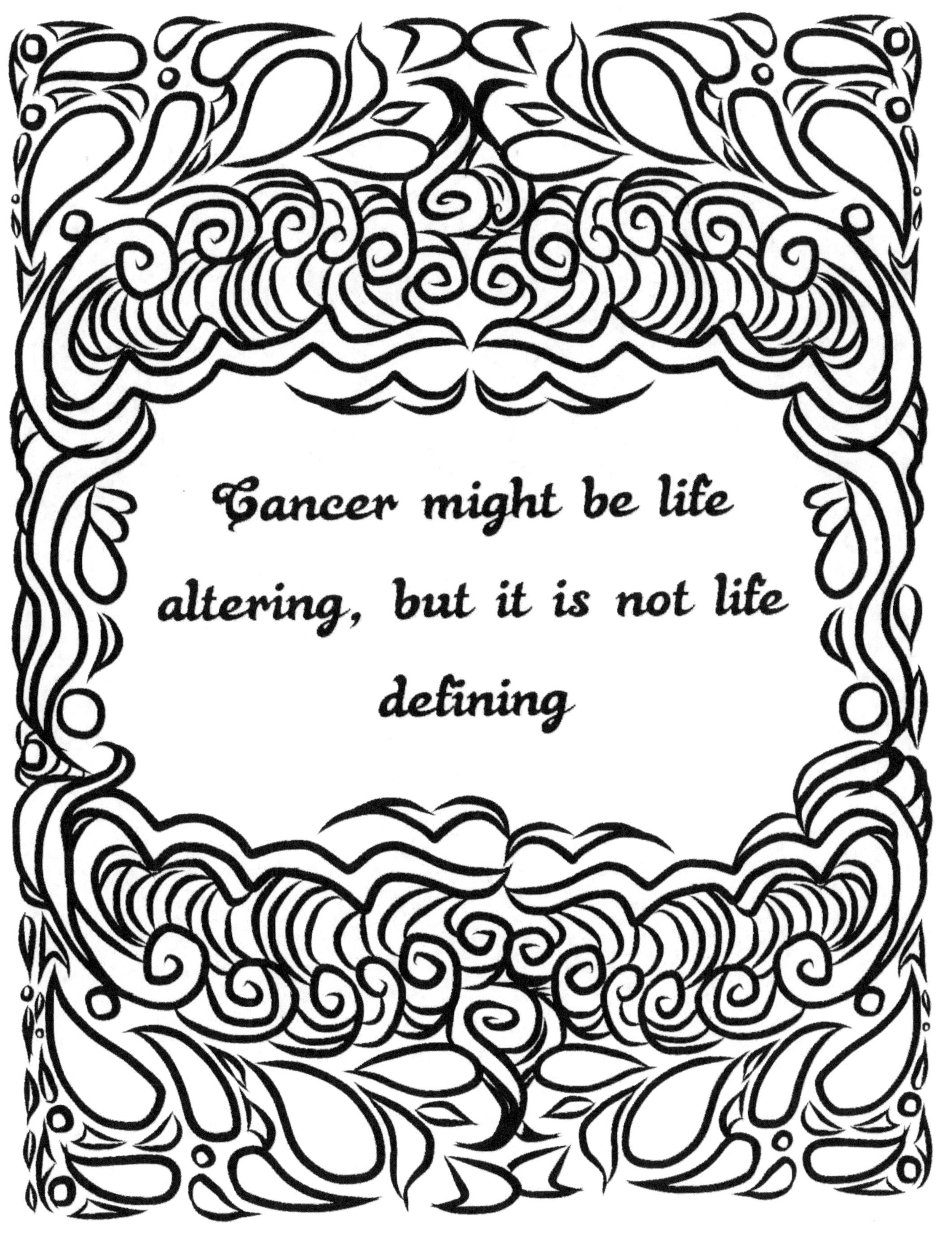
Cancer might be life altering, but it is not life defining

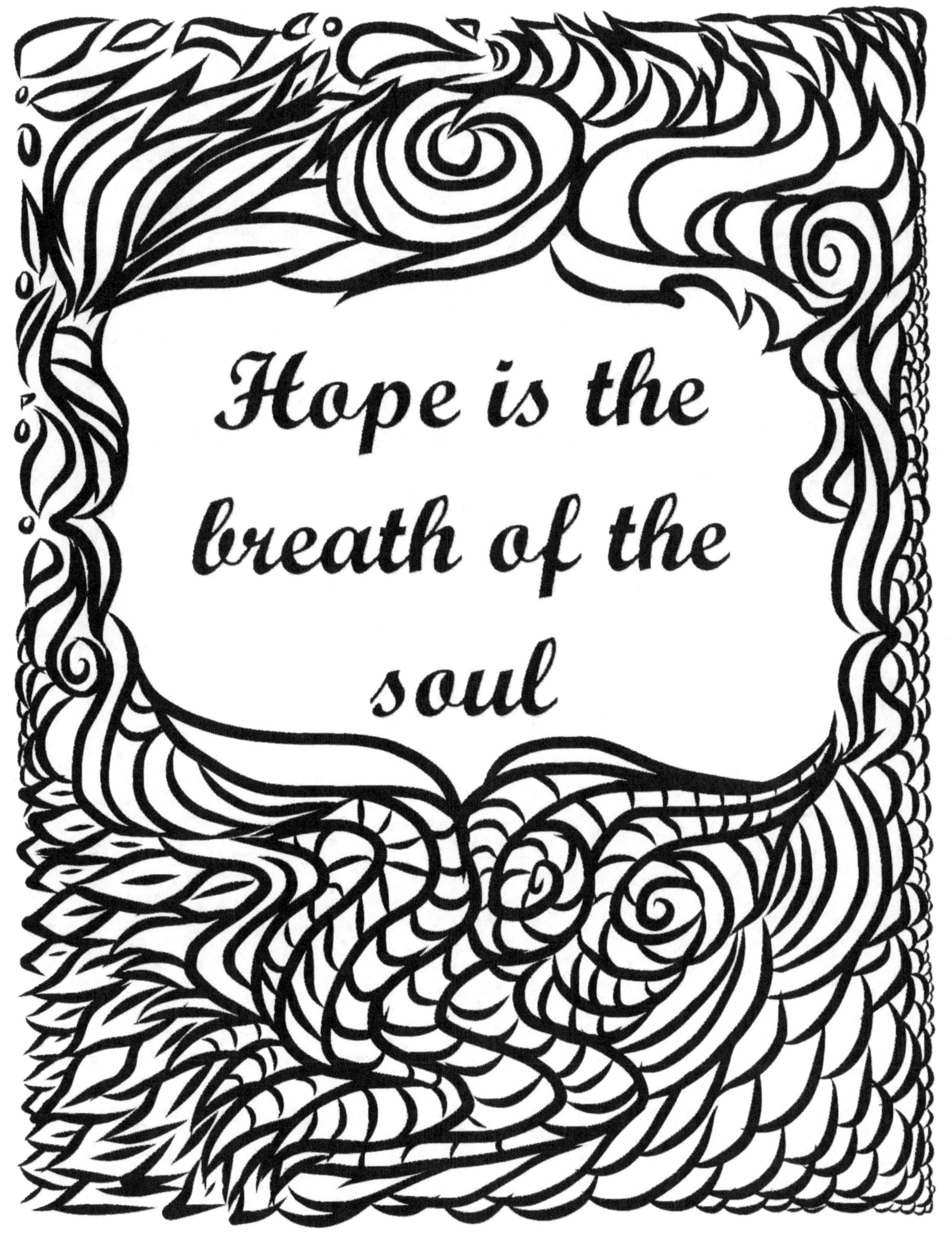
Hope is the
breath of the
soul

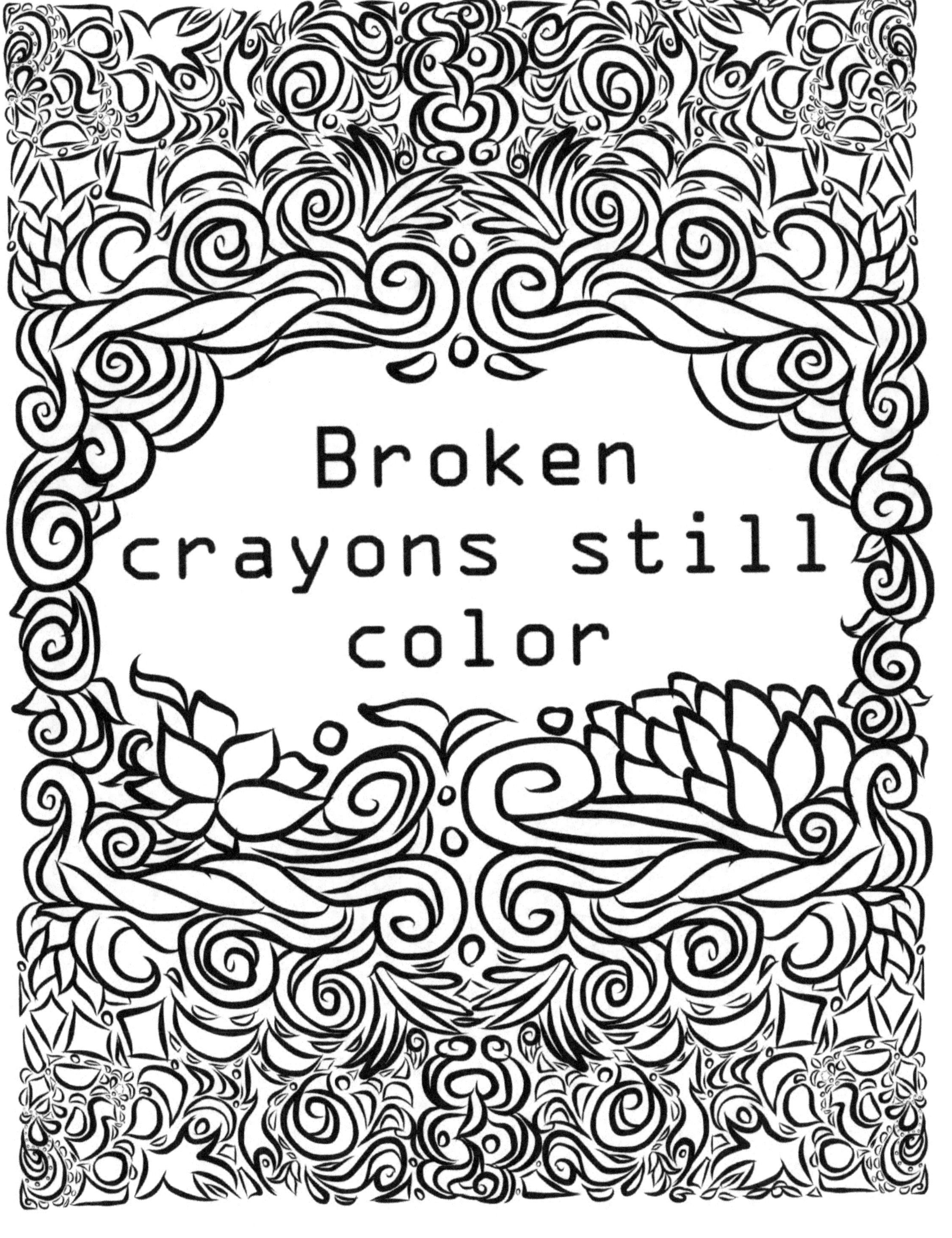

Broken
crayons still
color

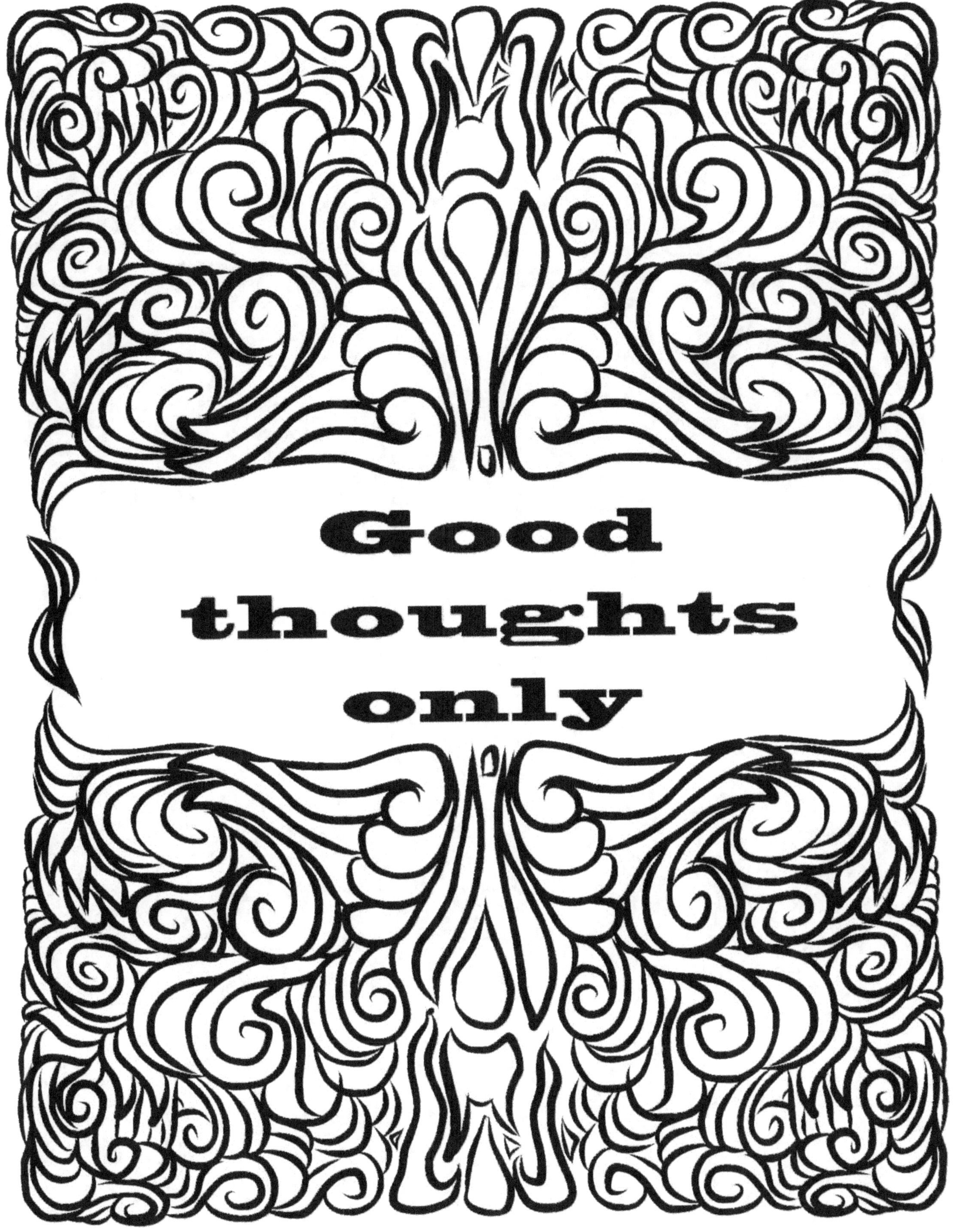

Good
thoughts
only

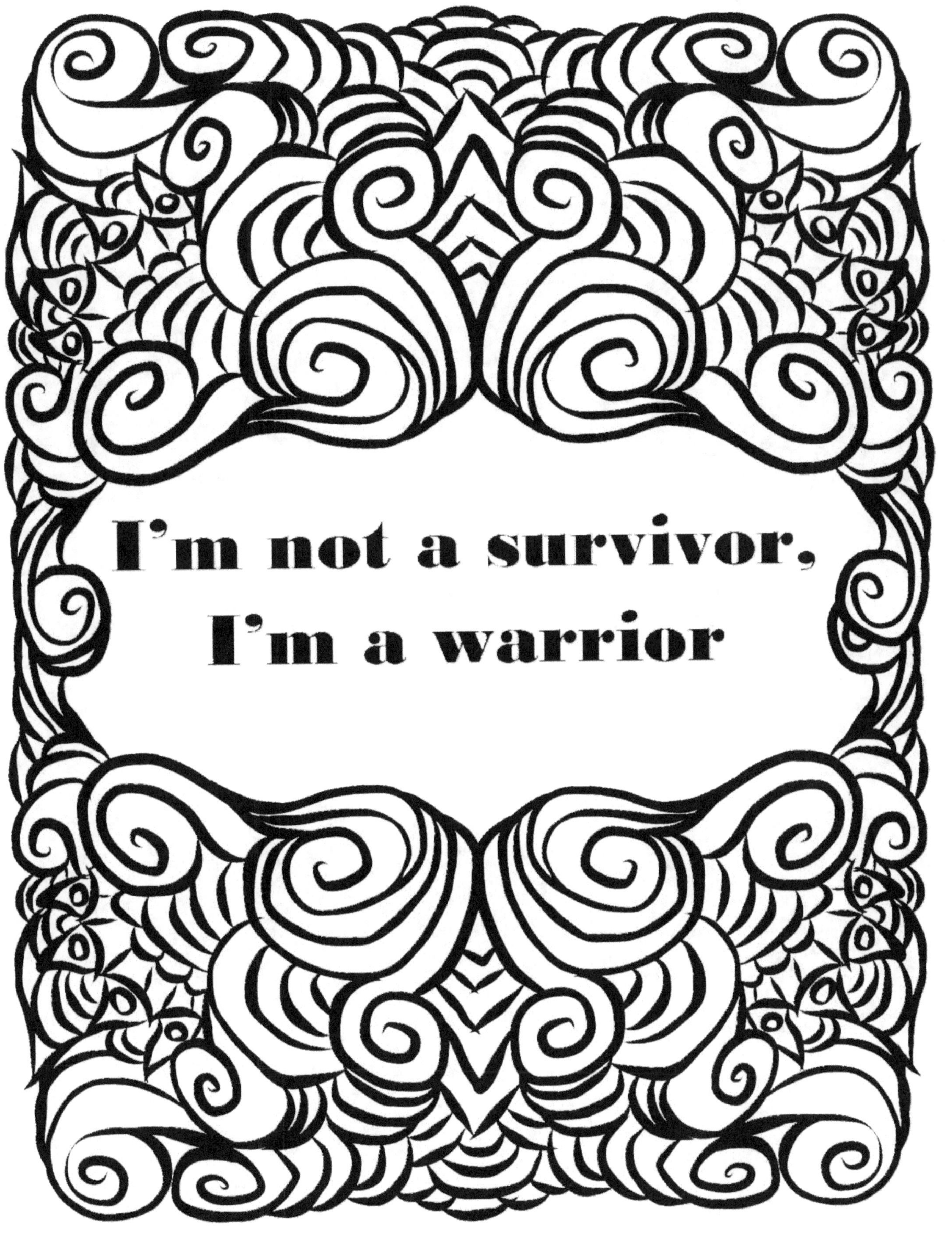

I'm not a survivor,
I'm a warrior

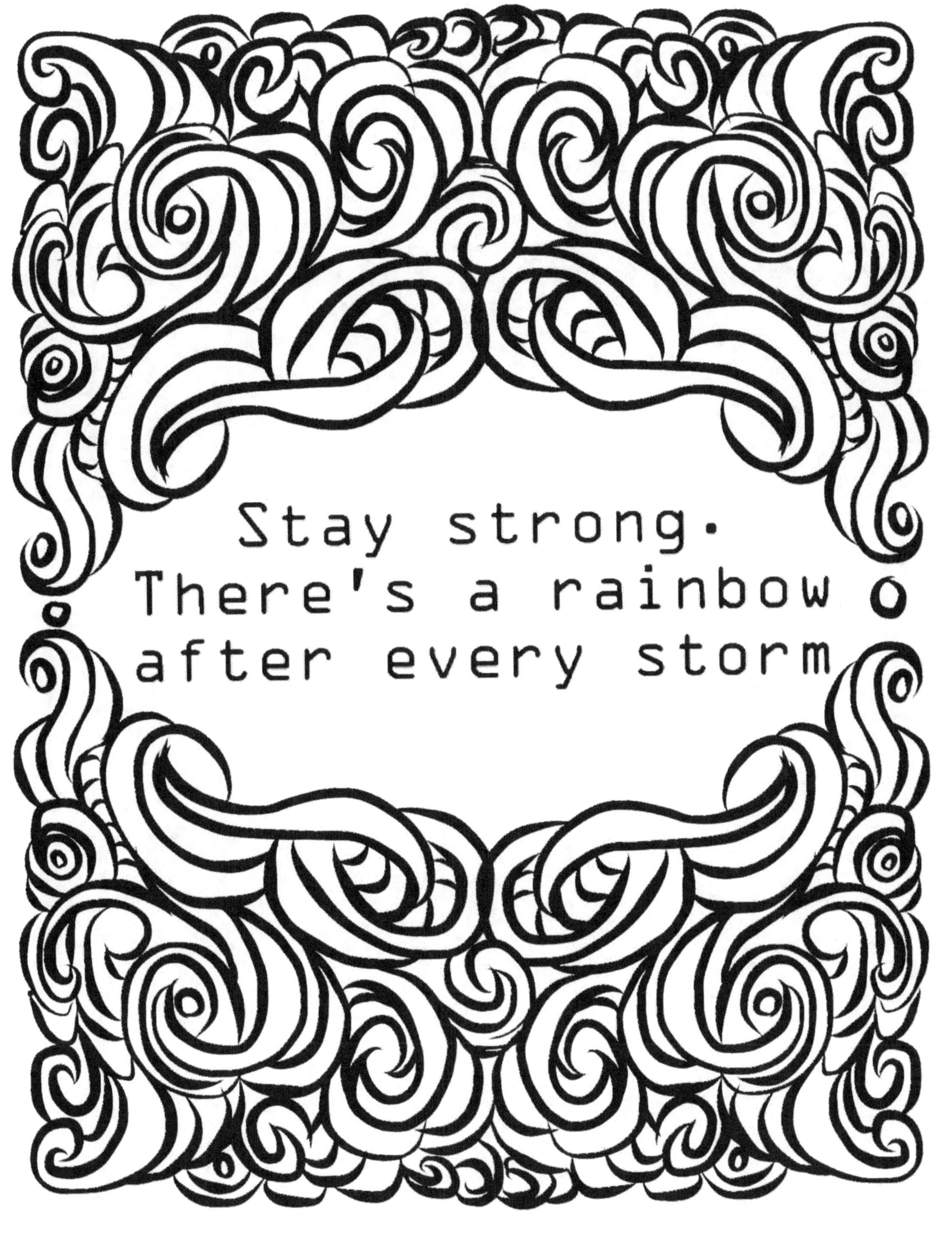
Stay strong.
There's a rainbow
after every storm

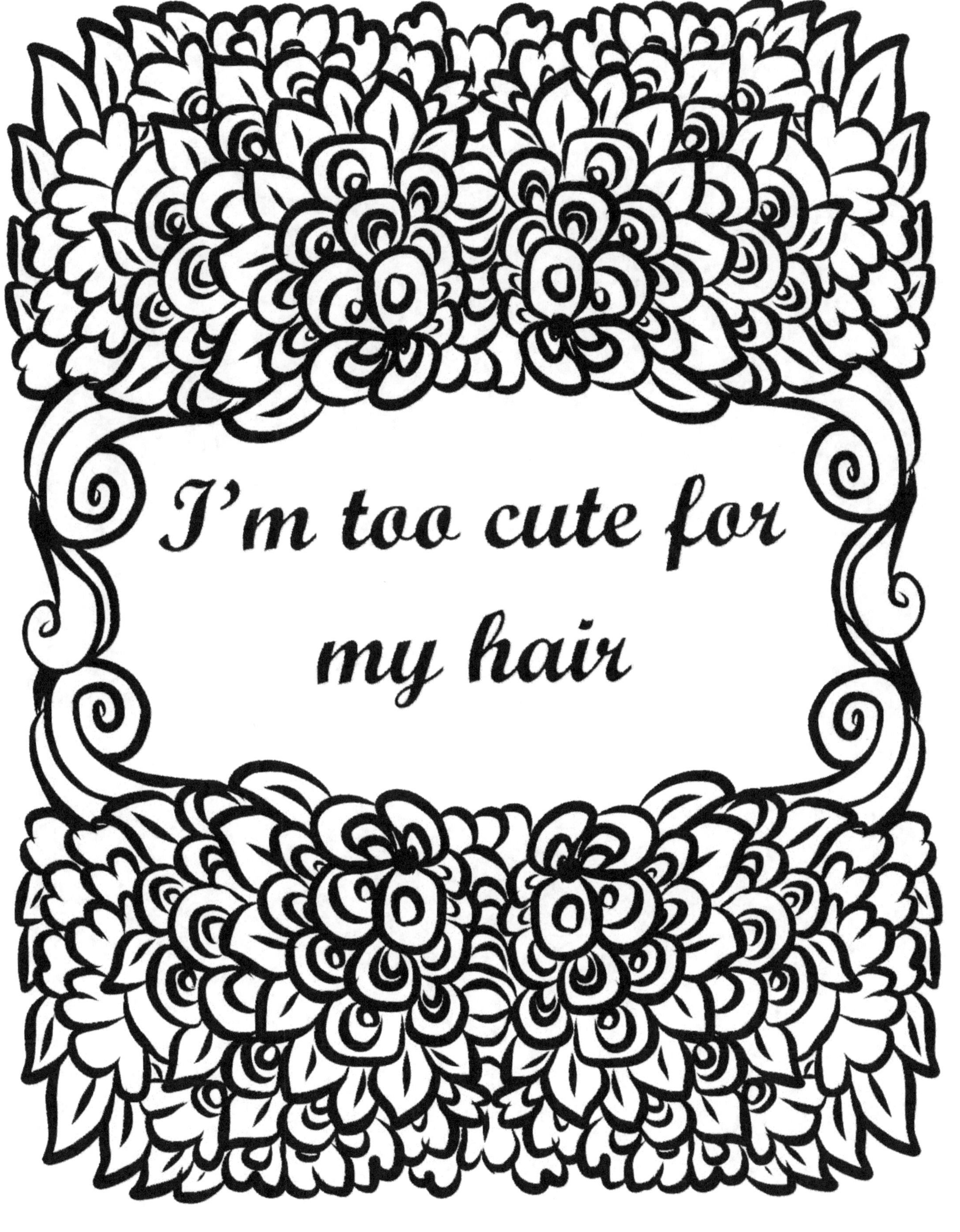

I'm too cute for
my hair

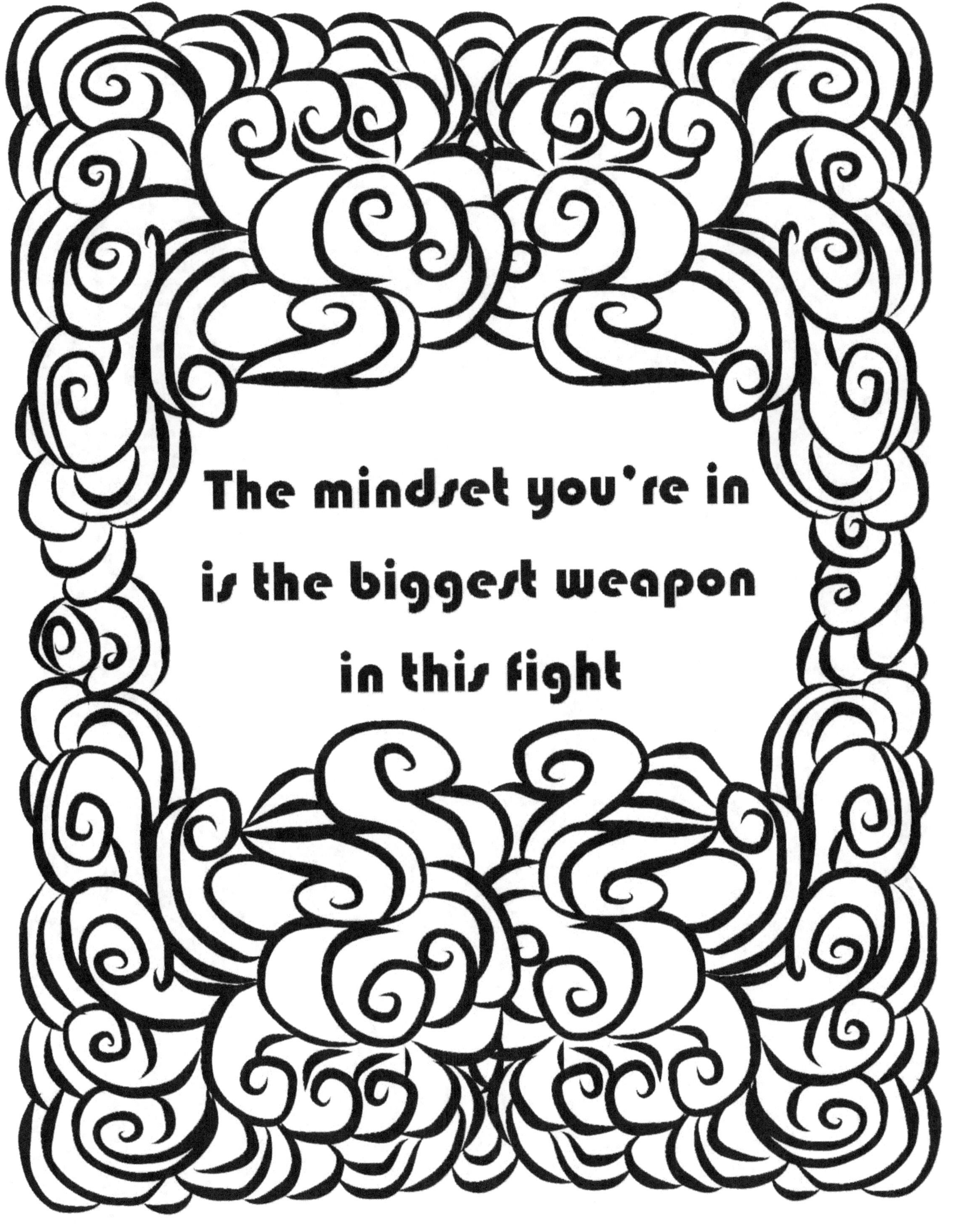

The mindset you're in
is the biggest weapon
in this fight

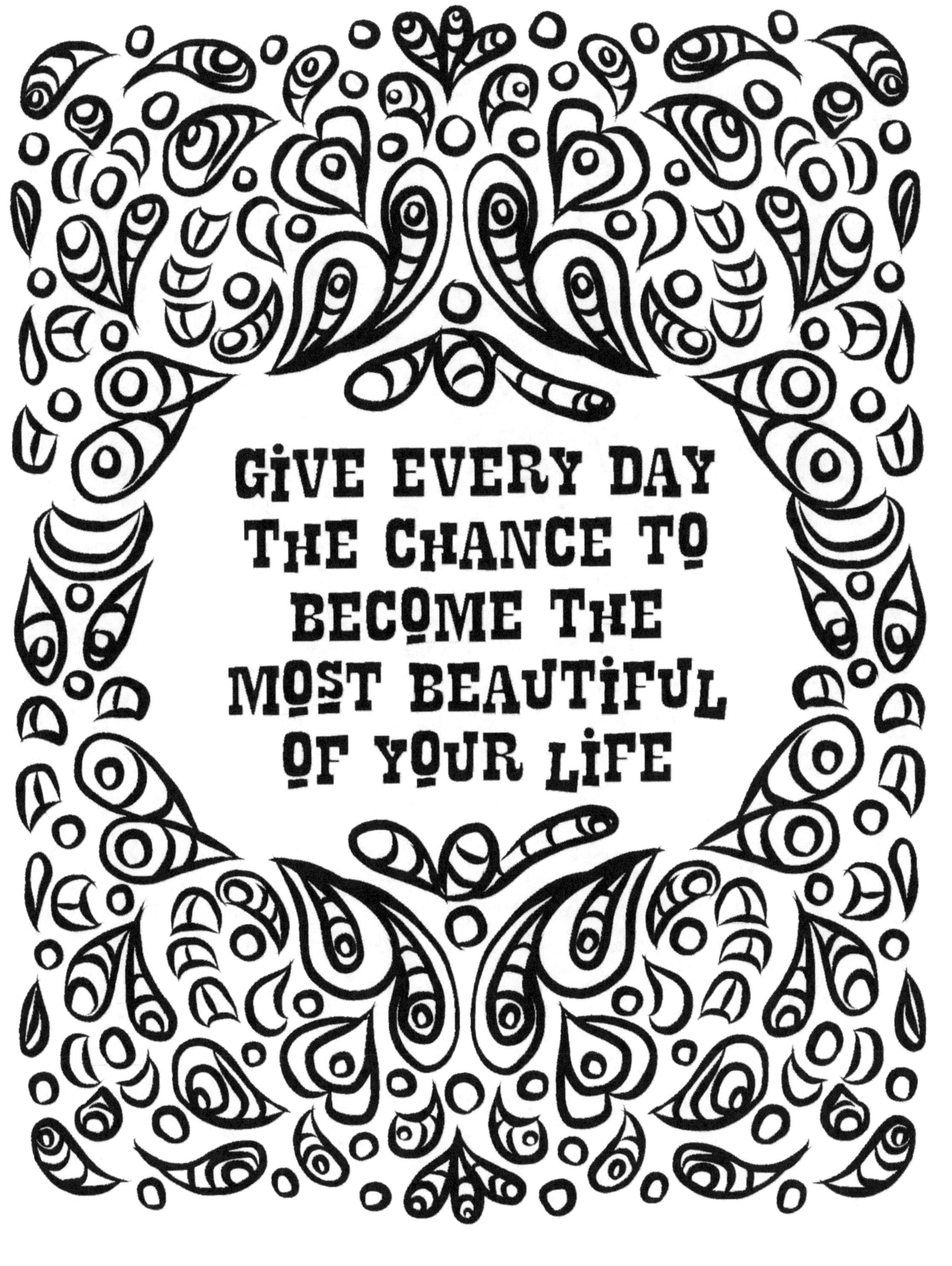

GIVE EVERY DAY
THE CHANCE TO
BECOME THE
MOST BEAUTIFUL
OF YOUR LIFE

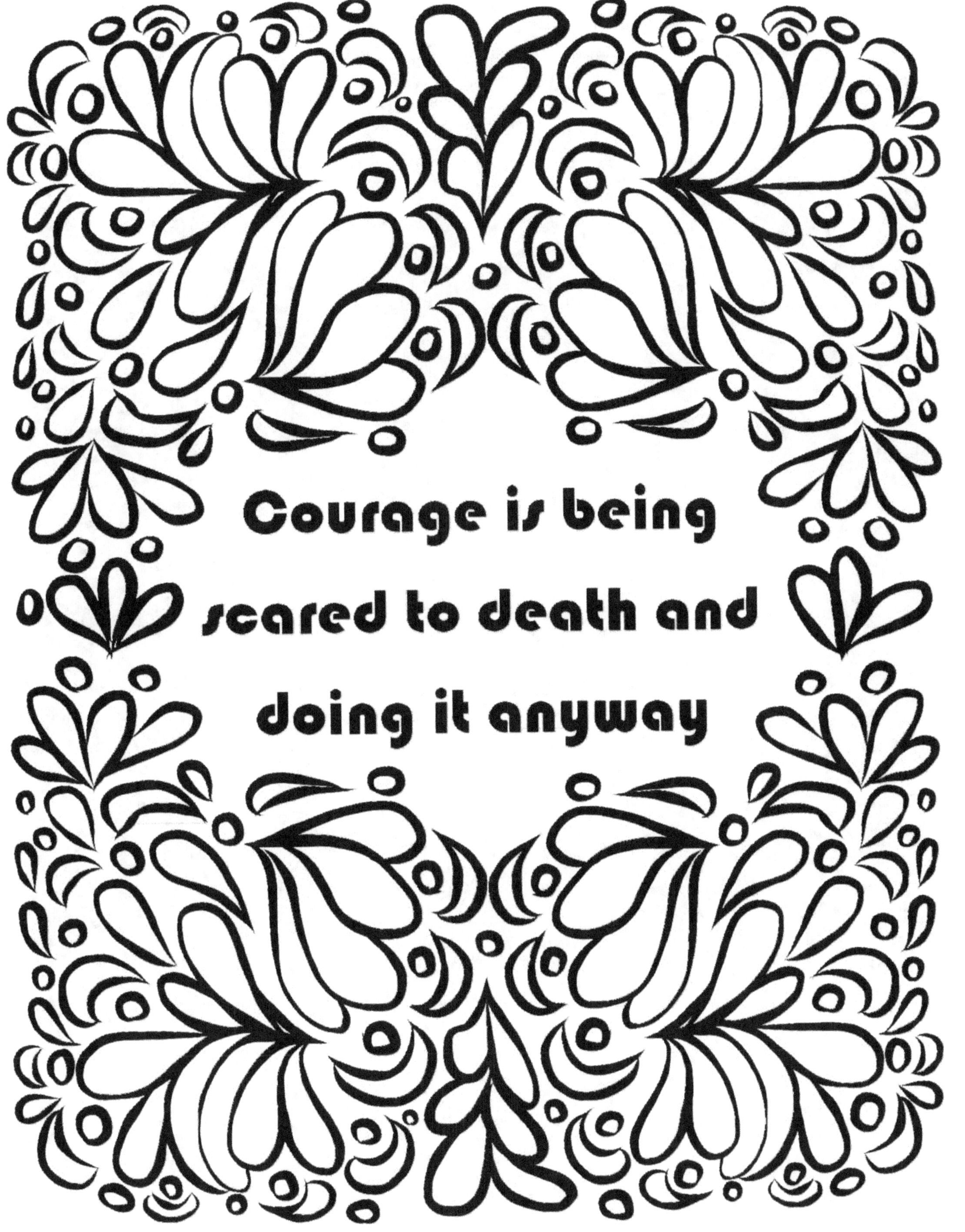

Courage is being
scared to death and
doing it anyway

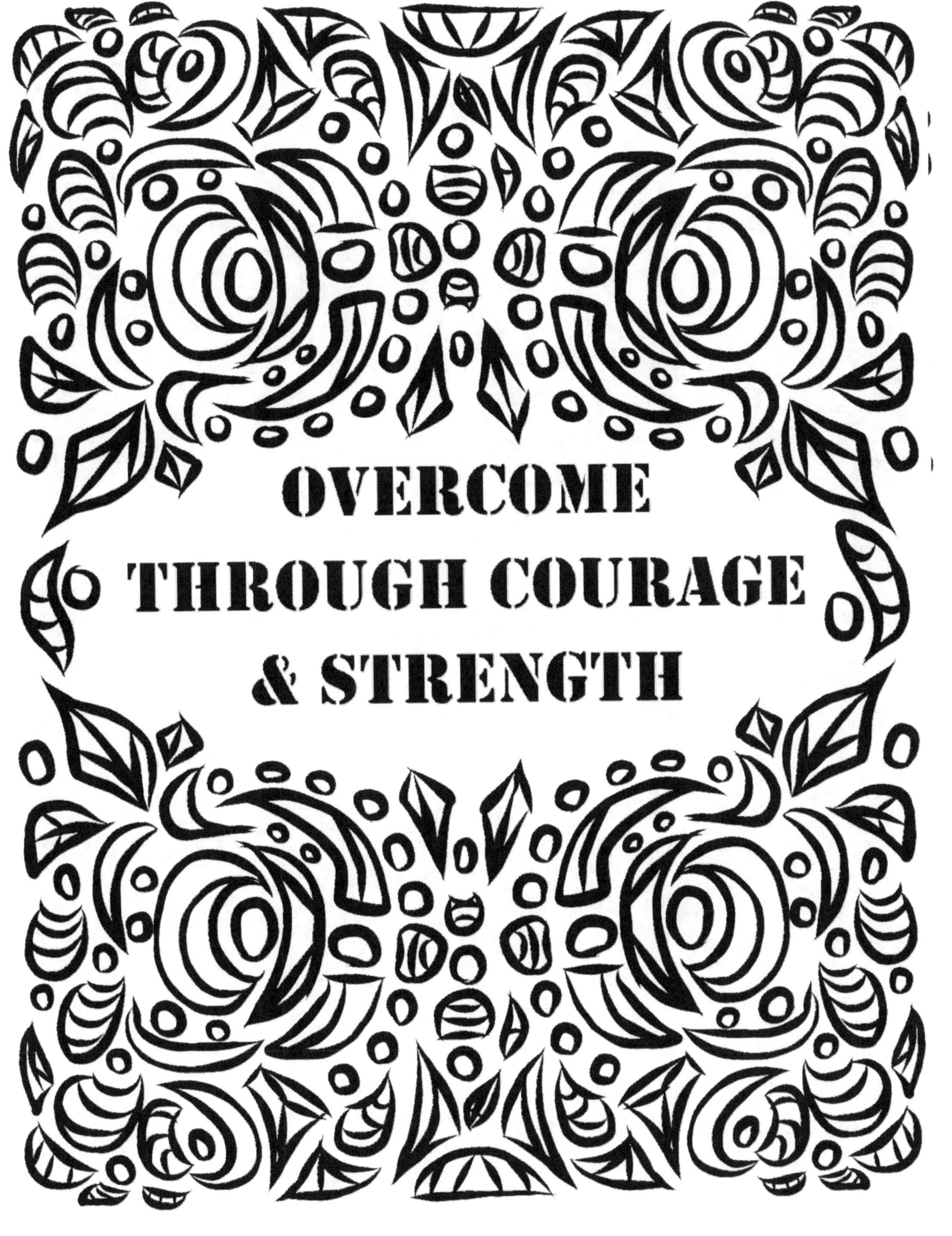

OVERCOME
THROUGH COURAGE
& STRENGTH

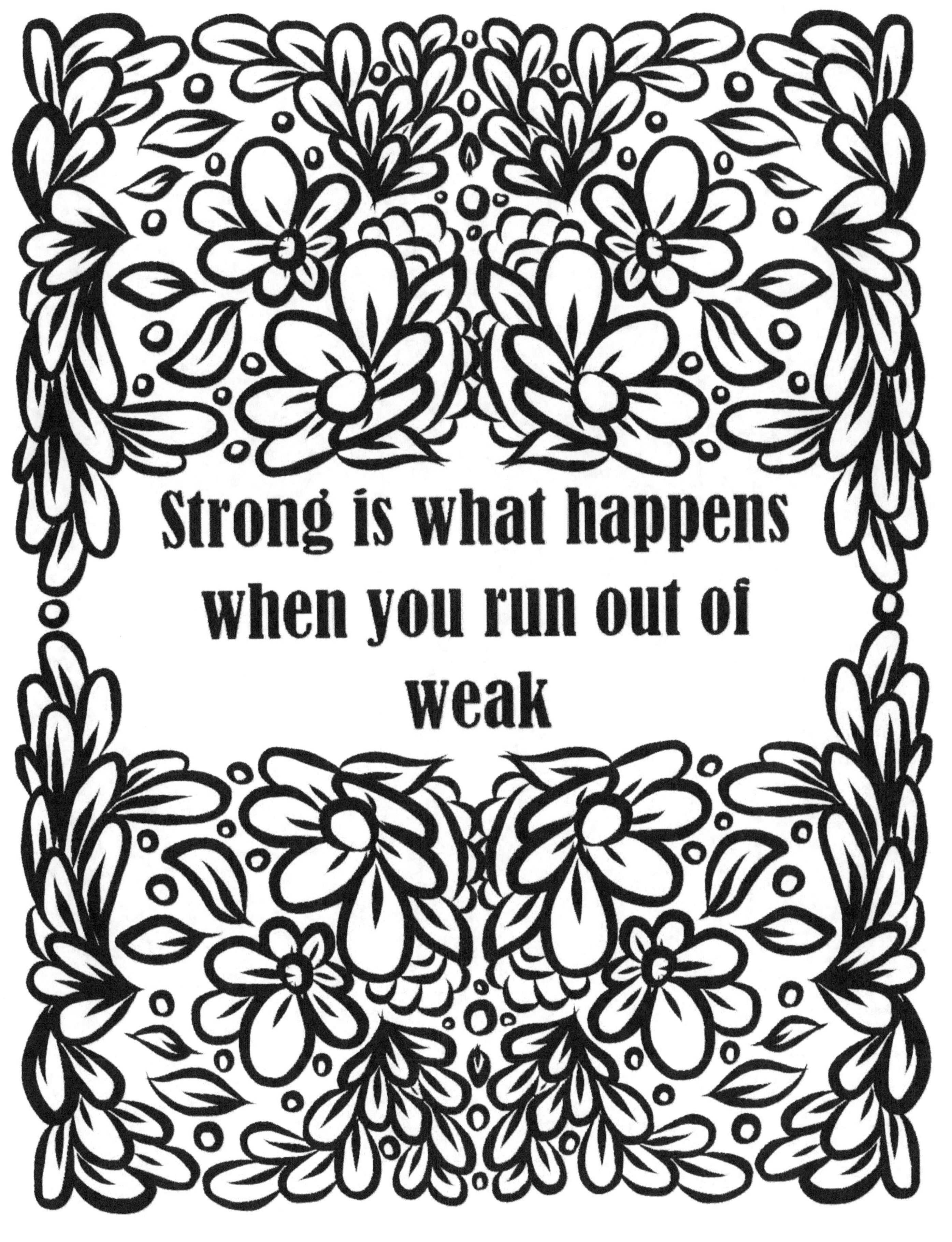

Strong is what happens
when you run out of
weak

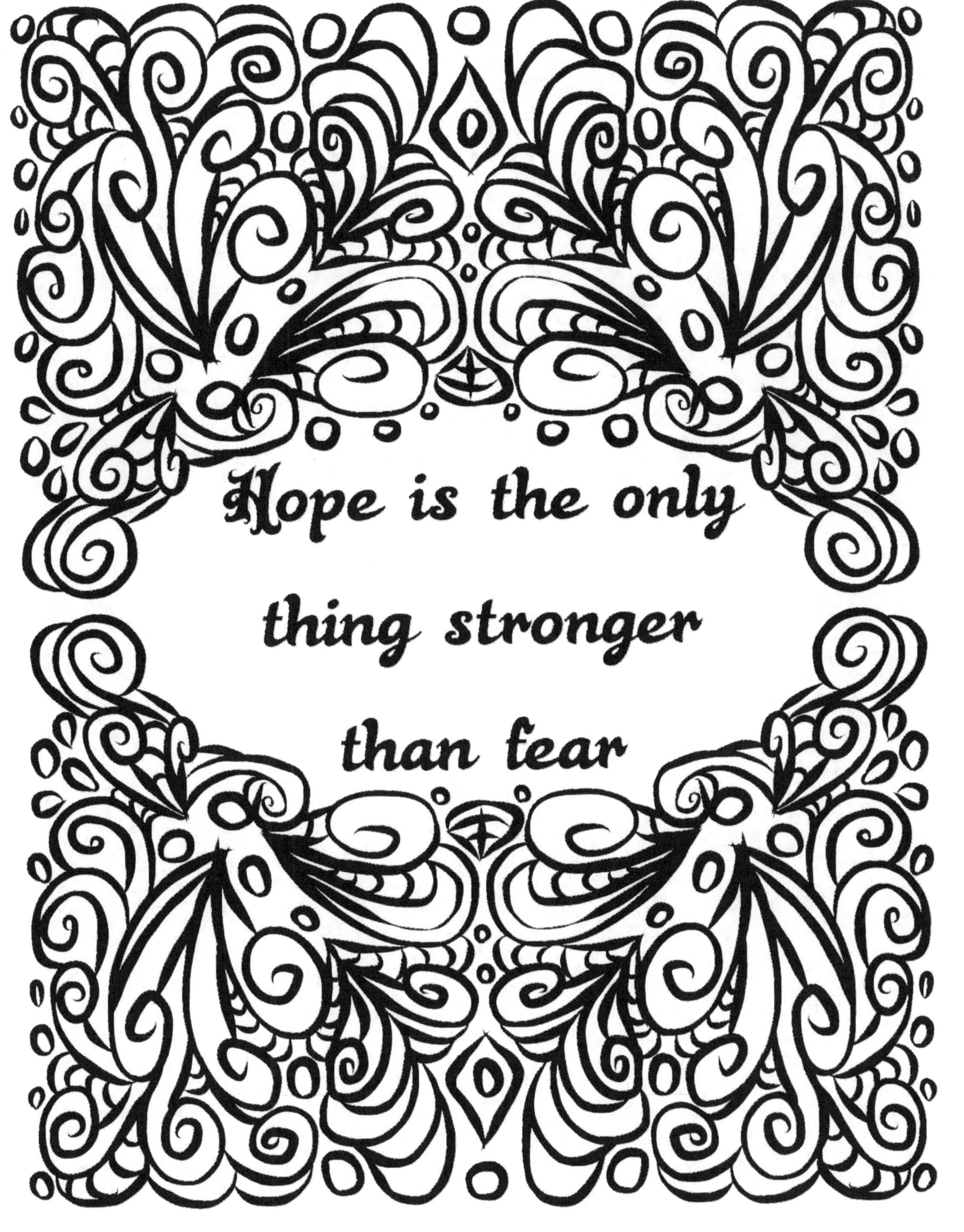

Hope is the only
thing stronger
than fear

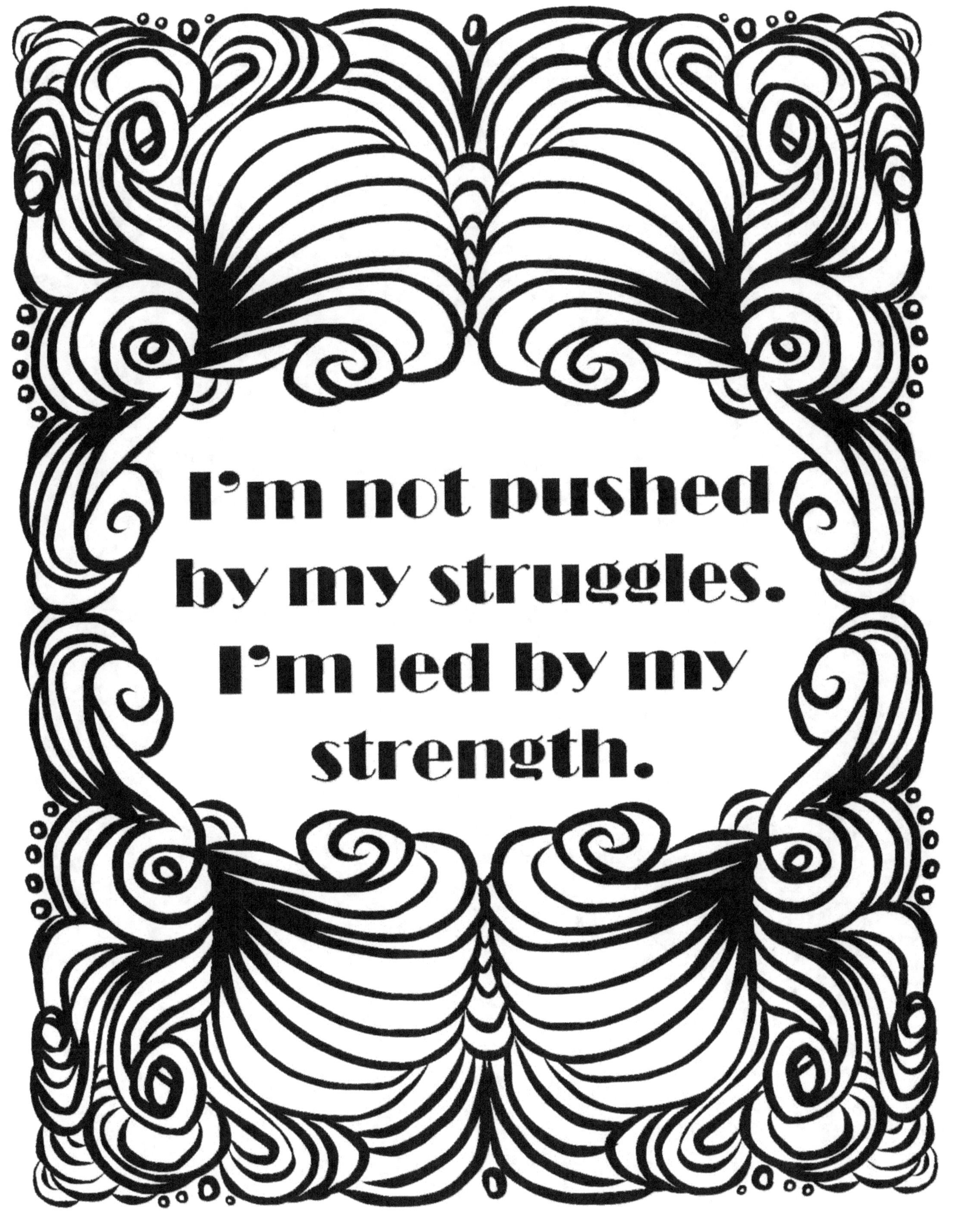
I'm not pushed
by my struggles.
I'm led by my
strength.

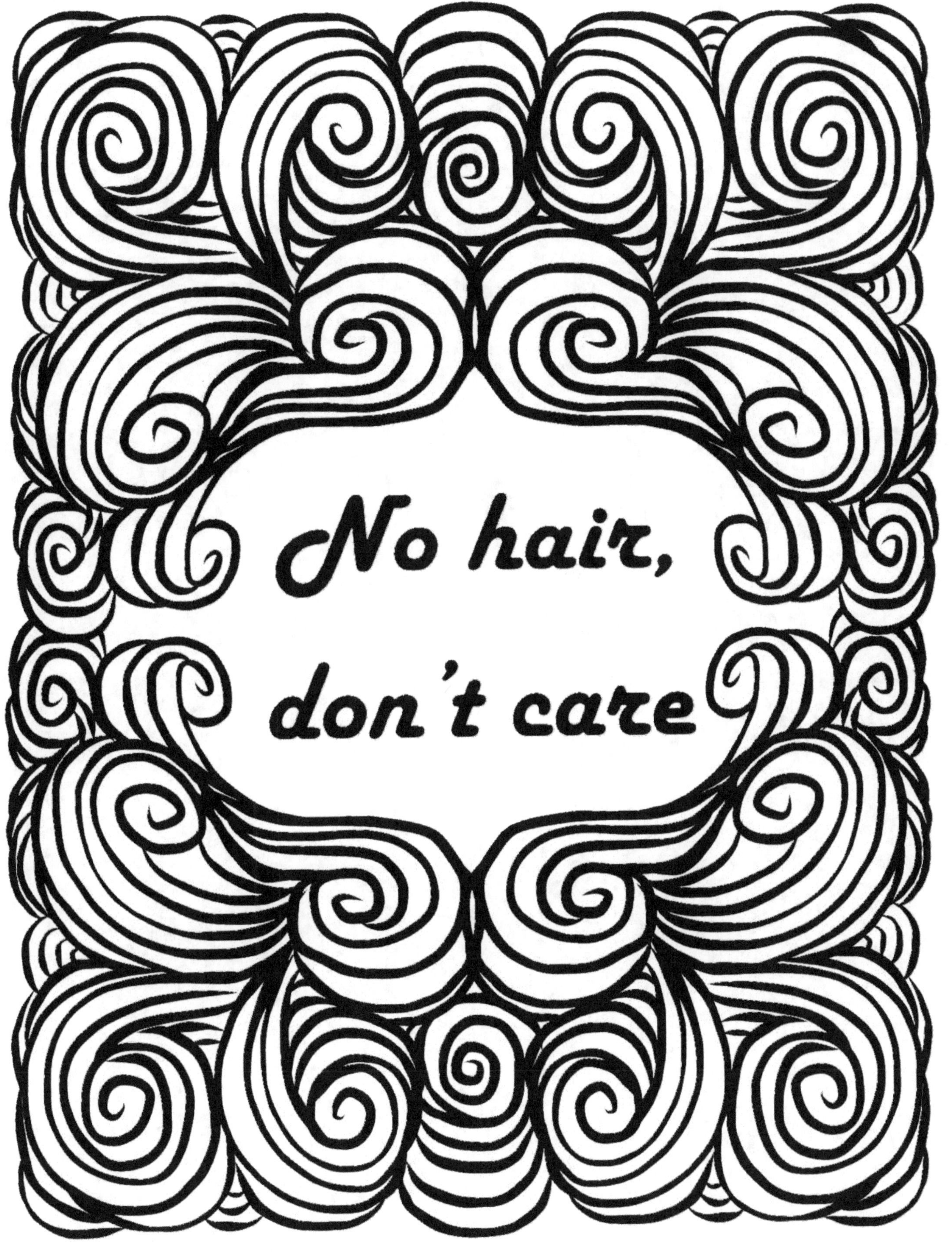
No hair,
don't care

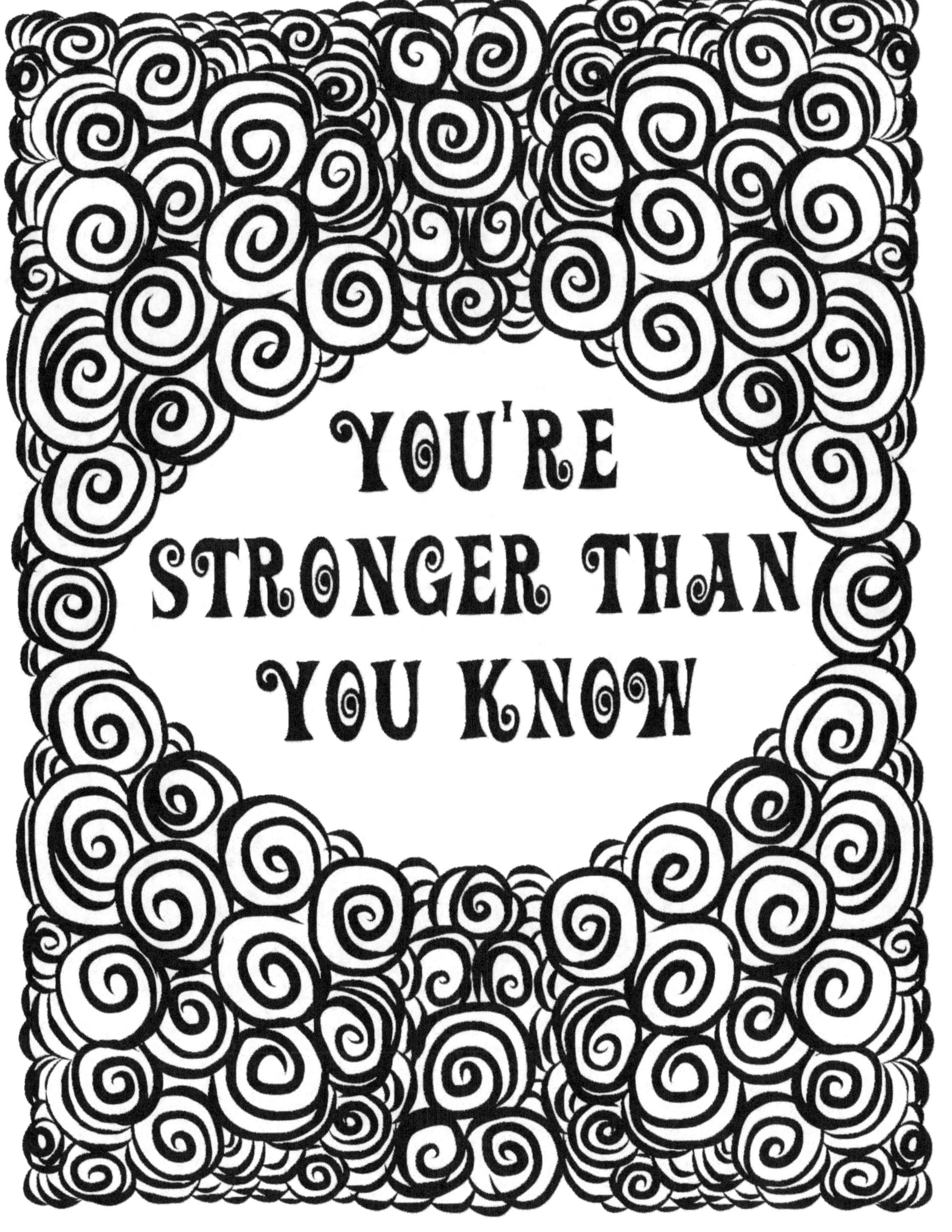

YOU'RE
STRONGER THAN
YOU KNOW

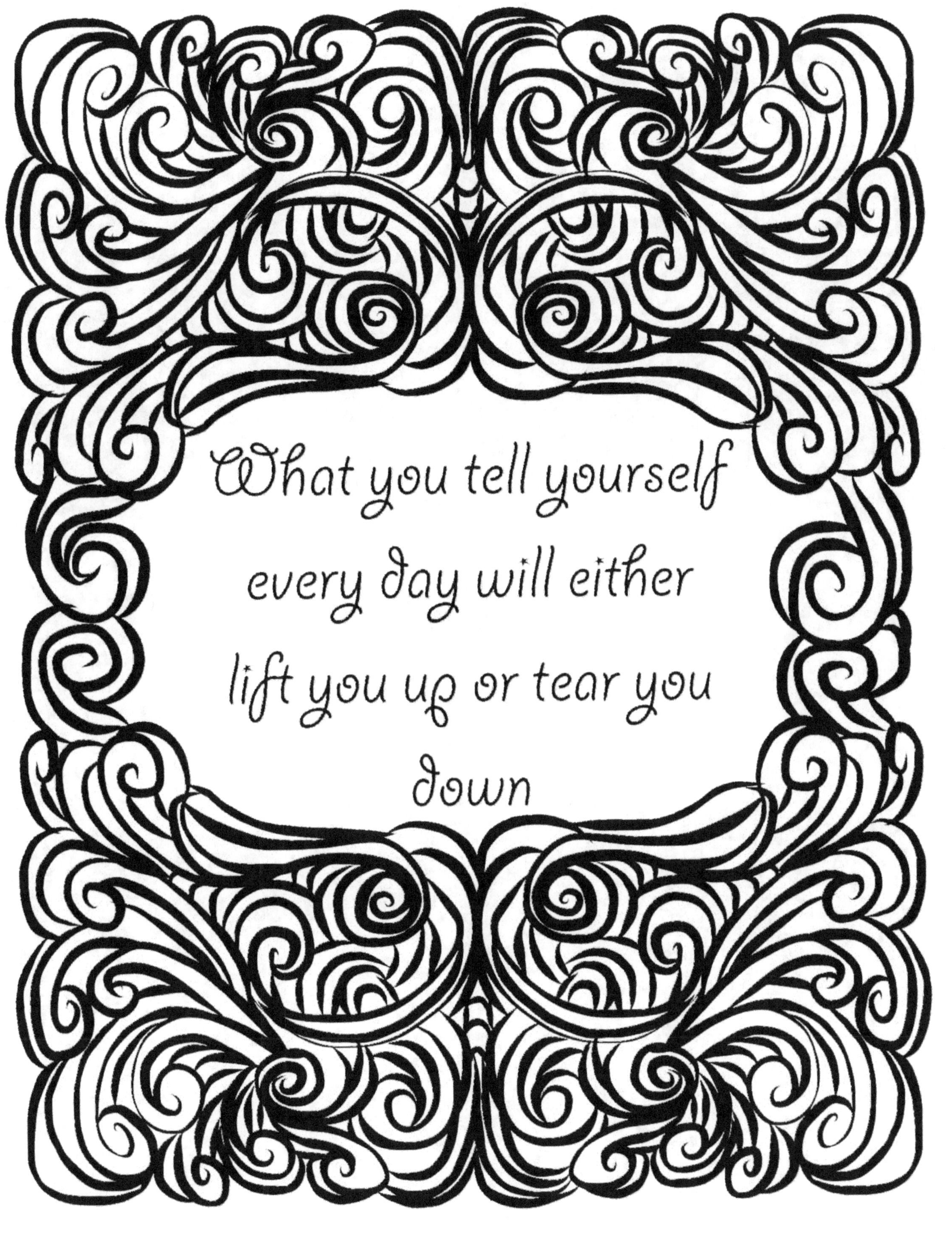
What you tell yourself
every day will either
lift you up or tear you
down

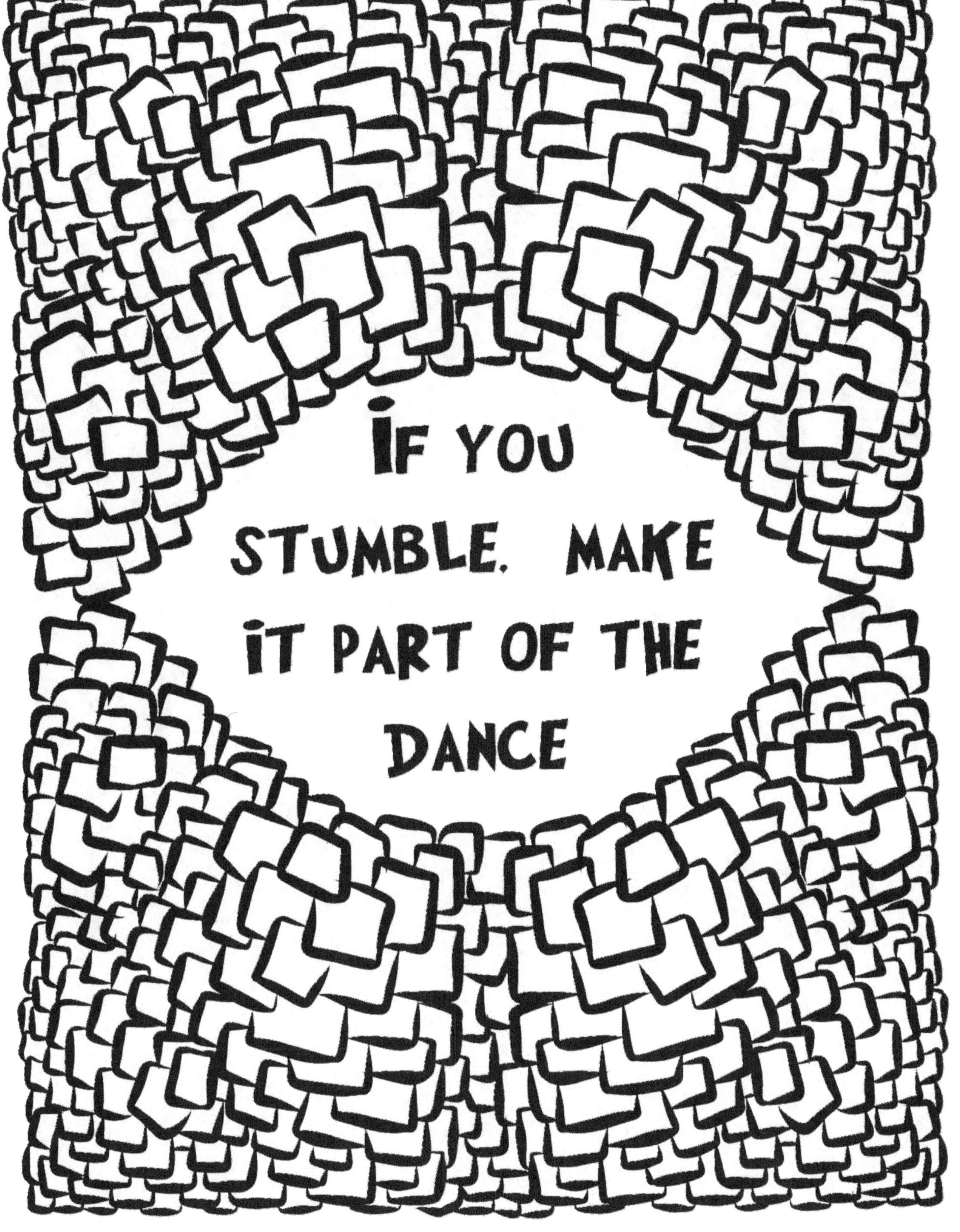

IF YOU STUMBLE. MAKE IT PART OF THE DANCE

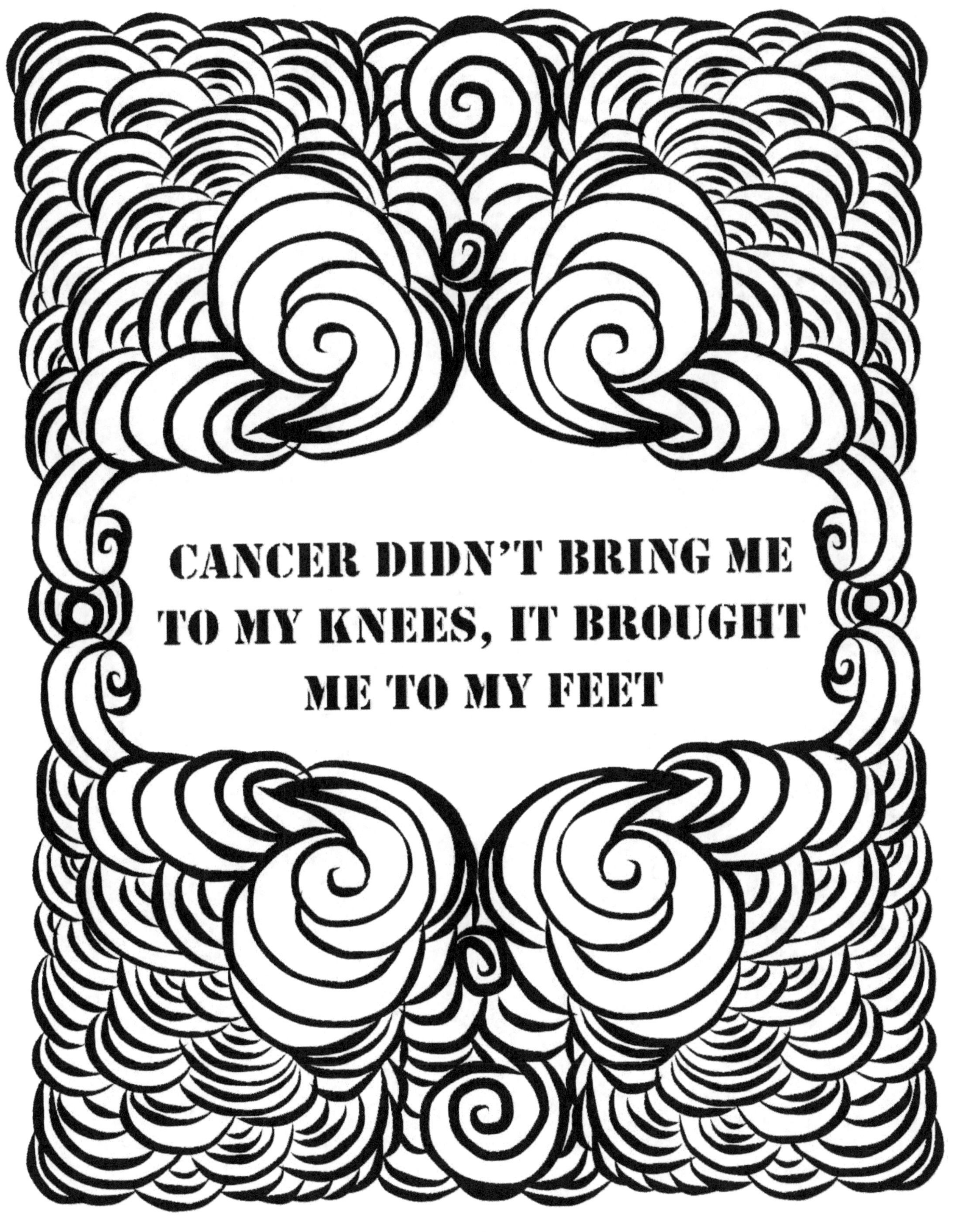
CANCER DIDN'T BRING ME
TO MY KNEES, IT BROUGHT
ME TO MY FEET

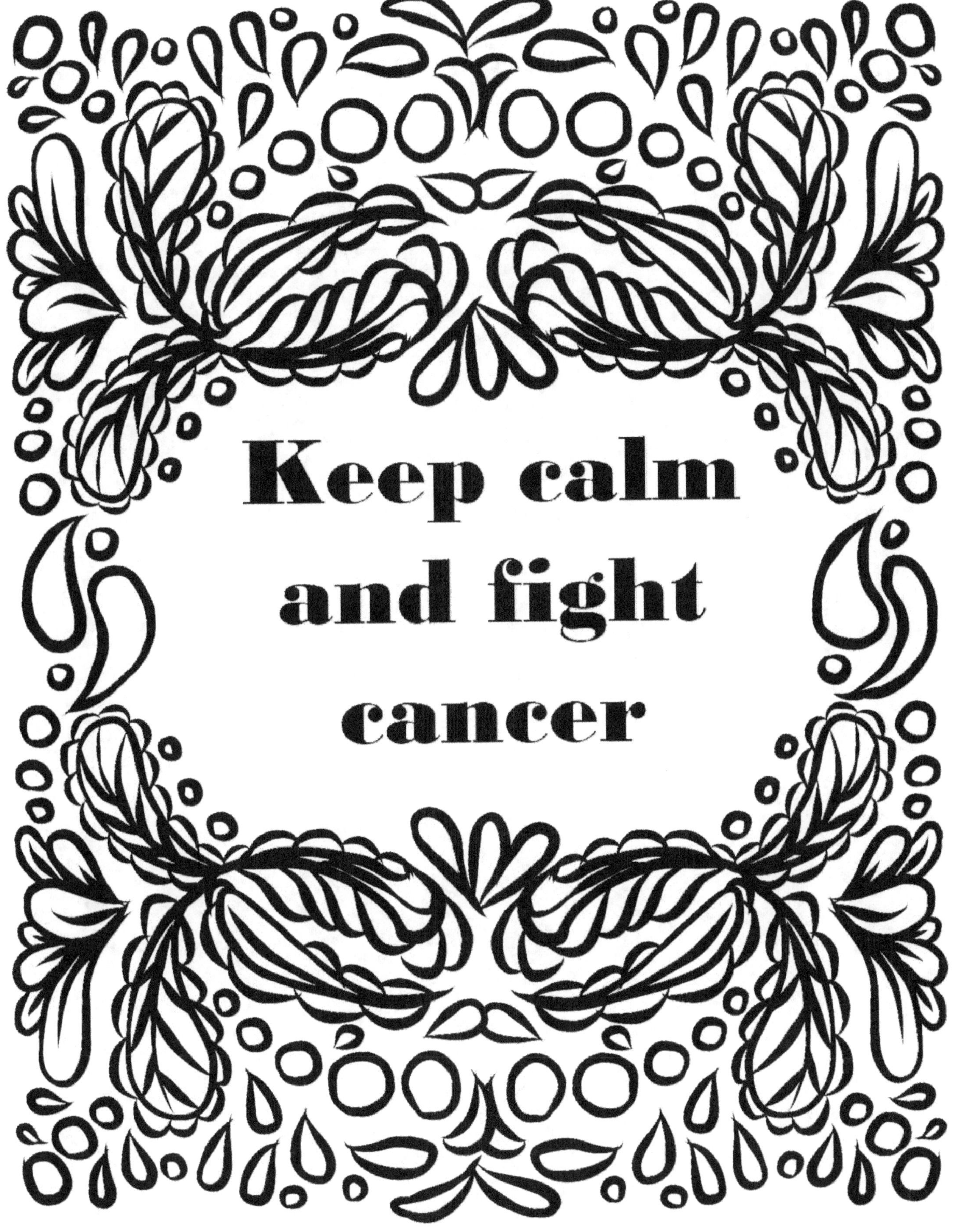

Keep calm
and fight
cancer

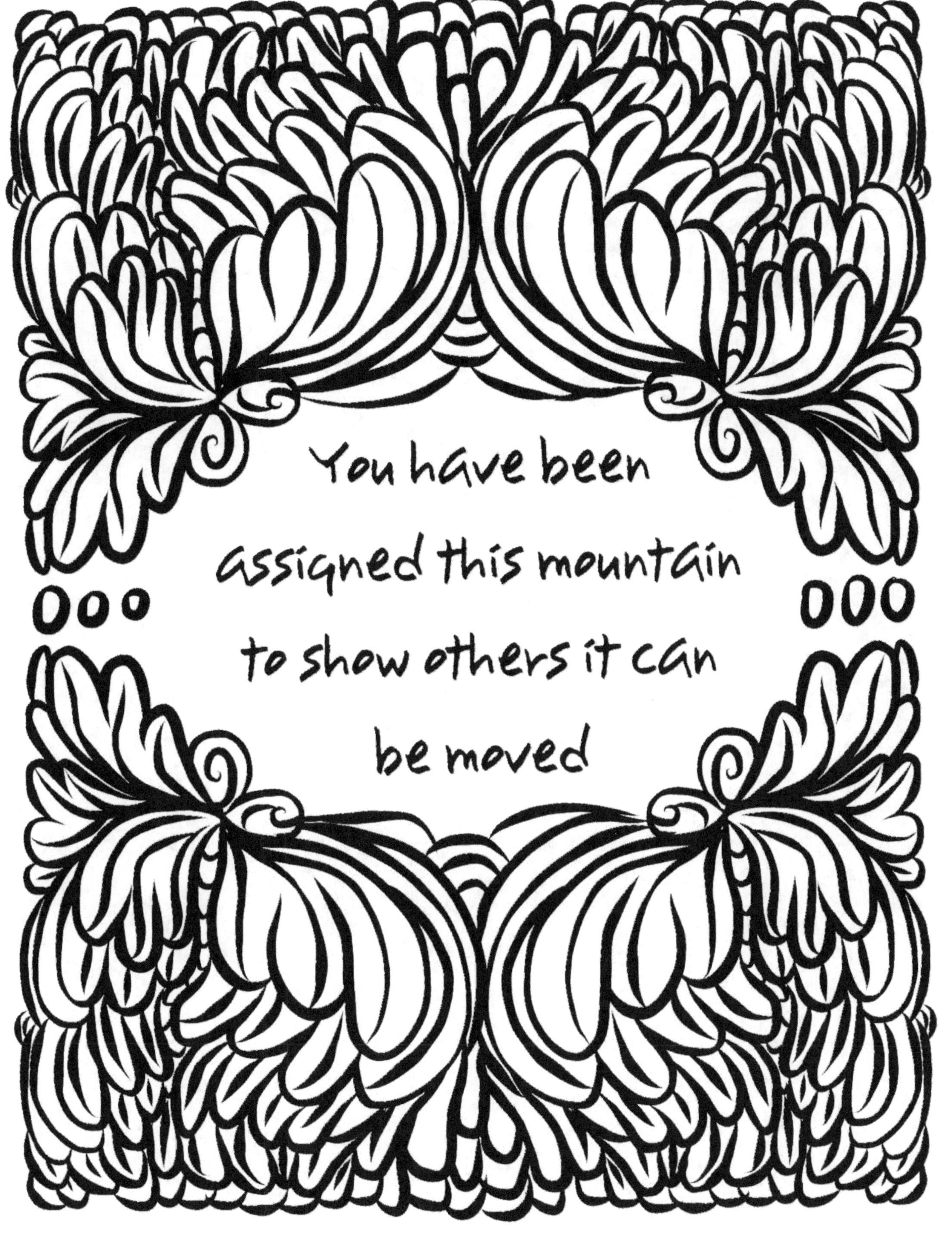
You have been
assigned this mountain
to show others it can
be moved

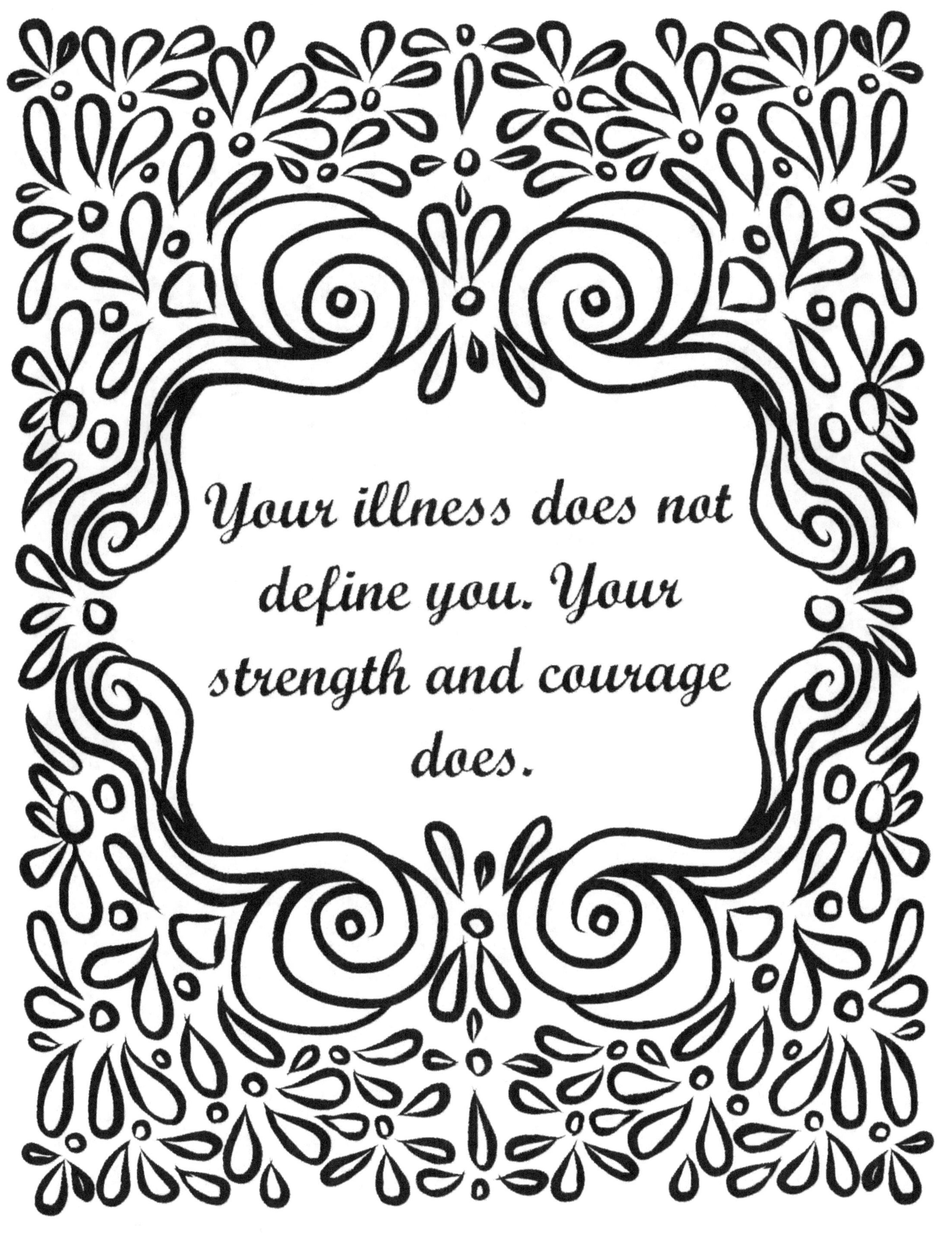

Your illness does not define you. Your strength and courage does.

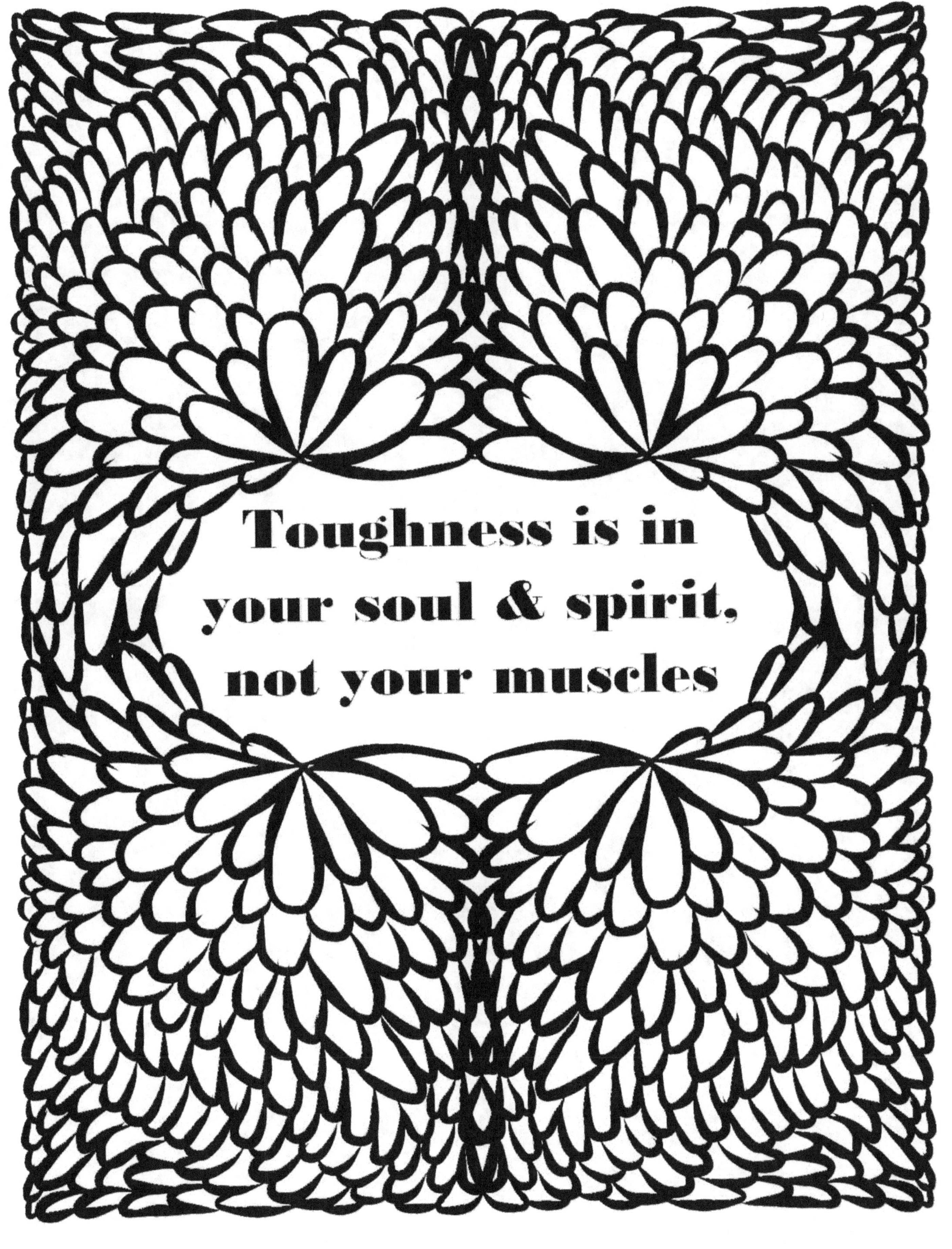
Toughness is in
your soul & spirit,
not your muscles

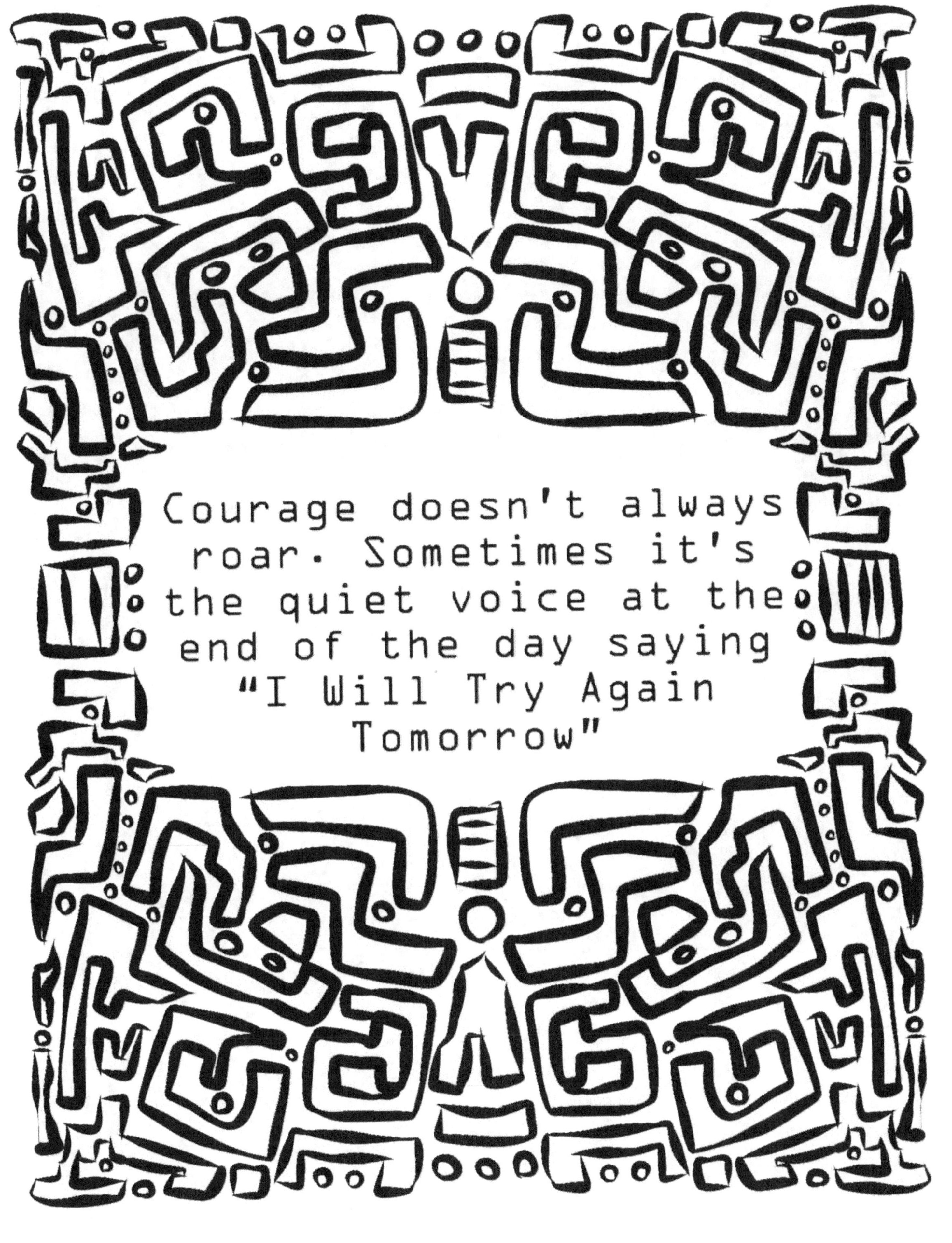

Courage doesn't always roar. Sometimes it's the quiet voice at the end of the day saying "I Will Try Again Tomorrow"

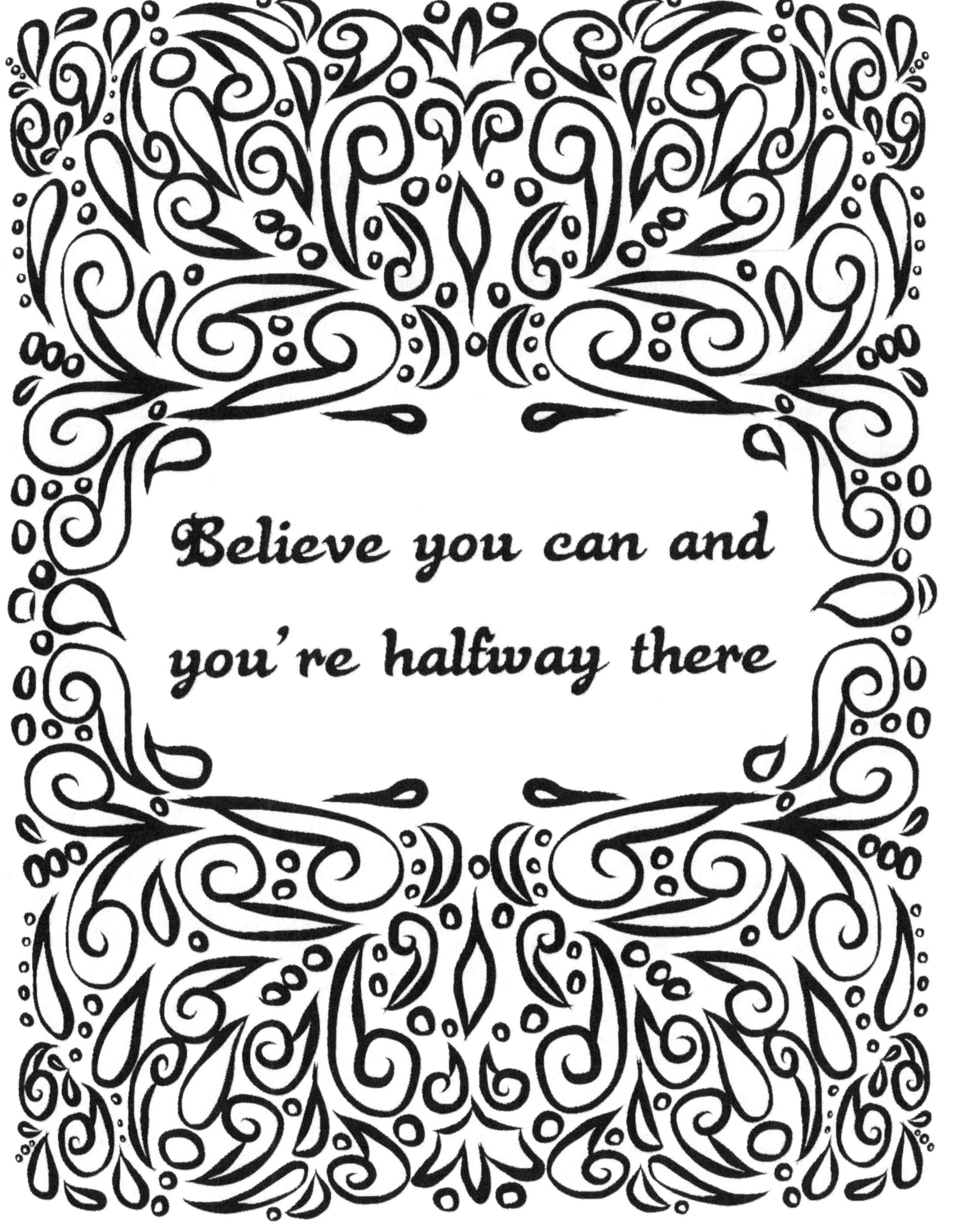

Believe you can and
you're halfway there

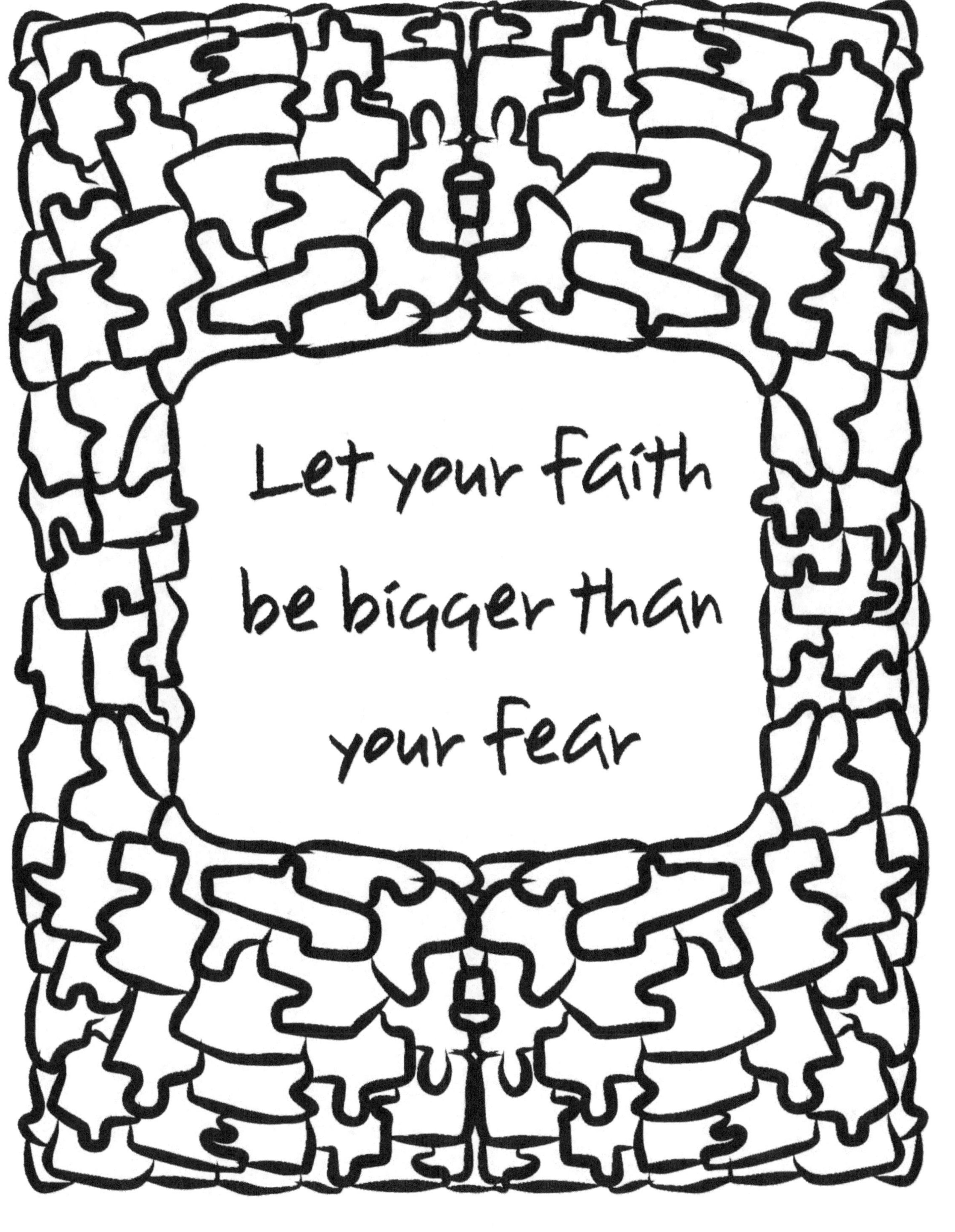

Let your faith
be bigger than
your fear

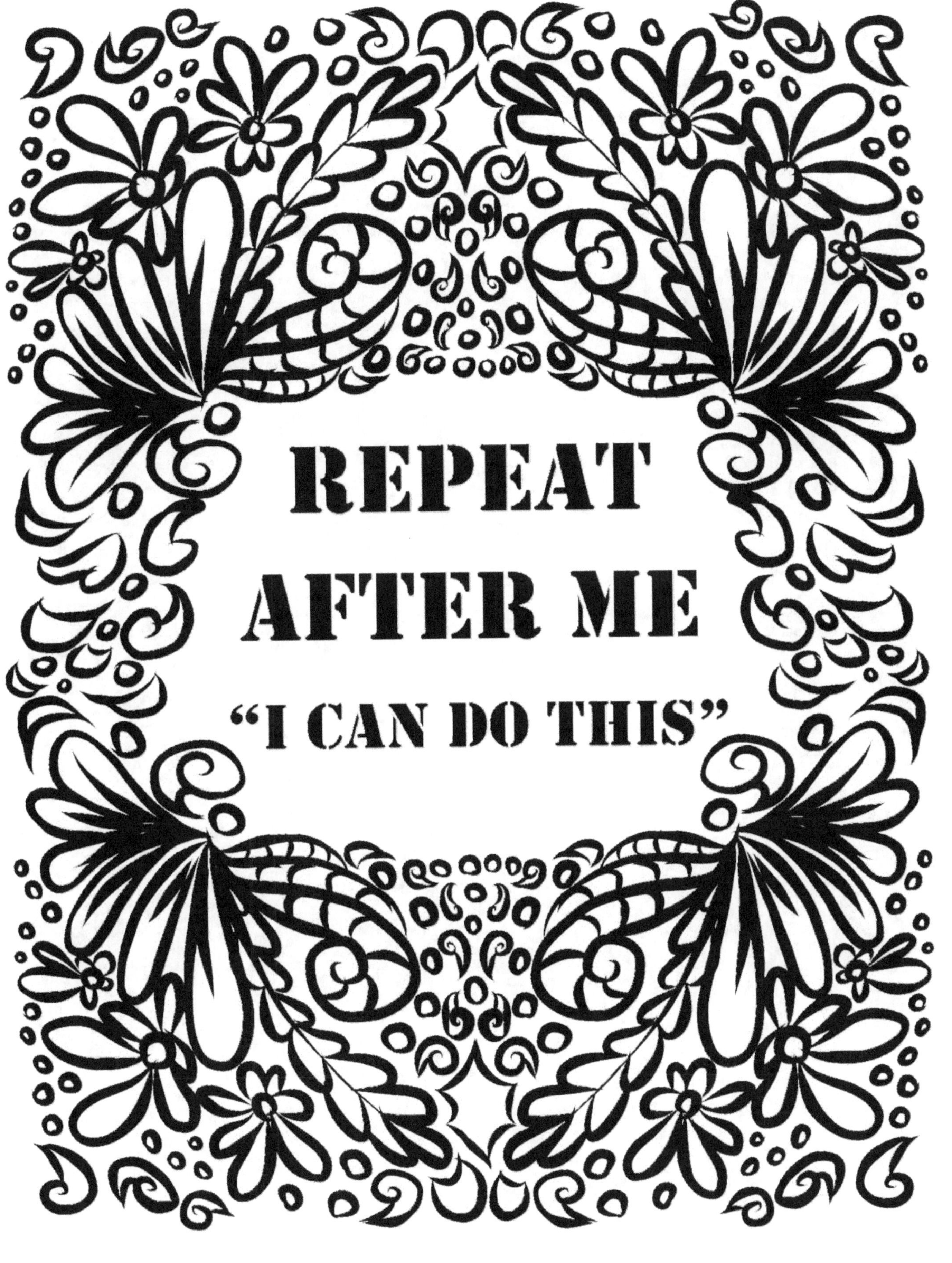

REPEAT
AFTER ME
"I CAN DO THIS"

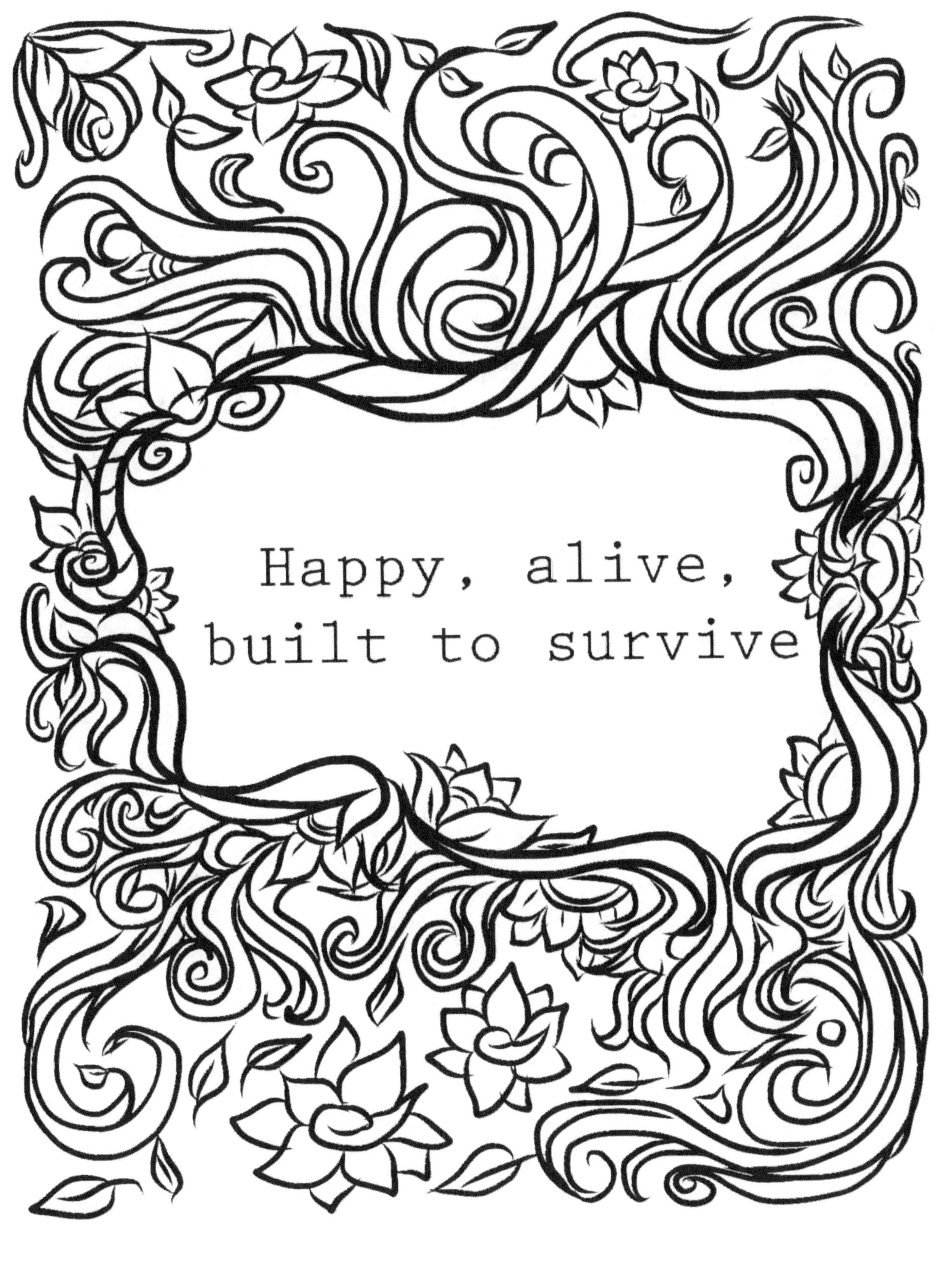

Happy, alive,
built to survive